AIDS
and Families

AIDS
and Families

Eleanor D. Macklin
Editor

AIDS and Families was simultaneously issued by The Haworth Press, Inc. under the title *AIDS and Families: Report of the AIDS Task Force, Groves Conference on Marriage and the Family*, a special issue of the journal *Marriage & Family Review*, Volume 13, Numbers 1/2 1989. Marvin B. Sussman, Journal Editor.

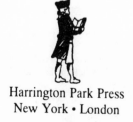

Harrington Park Press
New York • London

ISBN 0-918393-60-4

Published by

Harrington Park Press, Inc., 10 Alice Street, Binghamton, New York 13904-1580.
EUROSPAN/Haworth, 3 Henrietta Street, London WC2E 8LU England

Harrington Park Press, Inc. is a subsidiary of The Haworth Press, Inc., 10 Alice Street, Binghamton, New York 13904-1580.

AIDS and Families was originally published as *Marriage & Family Review*, Volume 13, Numbers 1/2 1989.

Cover design by Marshall Andrews.

Library of Congress Cataloging-in-Publication Data

AIDS and families / Eleanor D. Macklin, editor.
    p. cm.
    "Originally published as Marriage & family review, volume 13, numbers 1/2, 1989" — T.p. verso.
    Includes bibliographical references and index.
    ISBN 0-918393-60-4
    1. AIDS (Disease) — Social aspects. 2. AIDS (Disease) — Patients — Family relationships. 3. Family psychotherapy. I. Macklin, Eleanor D.
RC607.A26A345552   1989
362.1'969792 — dc20
                        89-32929
                        CIP

In dedication to

Gerald A. Brudenell, EdD
Associate Professor, Early Childhood Education
Florida State University
Member, Groves Conference on Marriage and the Family

who died October 6, 1987

and to his family and community
and all other families and communities who have lost
or will lose a loved one to AIDS

CONTENTS

ABOUT THE EDITOR

Eleanor D. Macklin, PhD, is Associate Professor, Department of Child, Family and Community Studies, and Director, Marriage and Family Therapy Program, at Syracuse University. She is nationally known for her leadership in the study of nontraditional family forms and in the field of family therapy. She is currently a member of the Steering Committee of the National Training Directors of the American Association for Marriage and Family Therapy, Chair of the AIDS Task Force of the Groves Conference on Marriage and the Family, and Co-Chair of the National Coalition on AIDS and Families. Dr. Macklin is a Clinical Member, an Approved Supervisor, and a Fellow in the American Association for Marriage and Family Therapy, and a certified sex educator and sex therapist with the American Association of Sex Educators, Counselors, and Therapists. She co-edited *Contemporary Families and Alternative Lifestyles: Handbook of Research and Theory* (Sage Publications) and wrote a chapter on nontraditional families in the newly published *Handbook on Marriage and the Family*.

Preface

Putting together a preface is a curious kind of job—written, as it is, after the fact. That gives it all the benefits of hindsight, of course; yet it also seems to carry with it a demand to be profound and to tease out the most important things the book has to say. The very notion of AIDS and the Family is paradoxical, I believe: we want to keep family in the AIDS picture, recognizing both its usefulness and its vulnerability; yet circumstances compel us to redefine the AIDS family in such a way that it no longer lends itself easily to conventional family therapy.

When the Groves Task Force on AIDS and the Family met in San Antonio, in 1987, to begin work on this book, 2 basic principles were set down. They were: (a) that we should consider family as the "Unit of Care," both the unit to receive care and the unit to give care; and (b) that we should define family broadly enough to include biological family, lovers and friendship systems, and also the "emerging families" of caregivers that often organize in response to a diagnosis of AIDS. In the months since that original meeting, I've come to respect and value those principles more and more; but I also believe, for the time being, they remain more ideal than real. In other words, I think these are ways to think about families that we can all reach for; yet I wonder how many of us, currently, can keep all those people in mind at one time.

I'm reminded of a time, several years ago, when I heard Ivan Boszormenyi-Nagy talk about something he called the multi-contractual ethic. At least that's the term as I remember it. He said he believed he had a responsibility to each member of a family, even those he'd never met—and that he had an obligation not to do harm to any of those. "Good idea," I remarked to a colleague, "but what a challenge to our more typical fault-finding attitudes toward family."

I don't think that most of us, even those of us who work with families on a day-to-day basis, can be that generous in our attitudes toward families. We tend, I think, to polarize — to see the family as good and one individual as having the problem, or to see our own client/patient as the victim of an inconsiderate or damaging family. Now as we try to go a step further and think of persons with AIDS and their families, we have to add several other groups of people to the equation — lovers and friends, friends of friends, volunteer care-givers, health care people. To my way of thinking, as the cast of characters increases the challenge to professionals working with families increases as well.

I'm most impressed with the Groves Conference, and with Ellie Macklin, who showed a remarkable foresight in calling a meeting where the subject of AIDS and the Family was discussed for perhaps the first time. Then they didn't stop with that, but they carried those ideas on into a National Coalition on AIDS and Families, and now this book. The tasks they took on were not easy ones.

As that meeting in San Antonio progressed, we all tried to keep family in mind, at the same time that we addressed specific AIDS-related issues. Sometimes that worked; sometimes it didn't. Since my own experience was with families and not with AIDS, I did more listening than talking. Then, I spent the next year or so reading and going to AIDS conferences, always wondering what my own role ought to be. Should I take a back seat because I could *only* talk about families, or should I pitch in and contribute whatever I thought would be useful? That's still a dilemma for me, as I think through what I have to offer at this critical juncture.

I come at this with a decided multigenerational bias — for a number of reasons. One is that I've been a family therapist for 18 years, working often with families in the midst of crises involving chronic or terminal illnesses. Another is that I'm a 60-year-old grandmother, looking at the world from a "Middle Generation" position. I knew, personally, two generations that preceded me, and now I know people in two generations of descendants. It seems silly that life should look so different from that vantage point, but it enables me to put myself in a lot of other people's shoes, so to speak. Also I have a different sense of how values and attitudes moved through the family, down to my generation, and I can speculate about the influence I have had and will continue to have on the generations that follow. What will I teach them, for example, by the way I behave in the face of this epidemic called AIDS?

My interest in my own family of origin began some 32 years ago, after the birth of my daughter—when it dawned on me that in my maternal line, at least, mothers dealt pretty well with their sons but they didn't have much idea at all what to do with daughters. Between mothers and daughters—for at least the three generations I knew about—there was typically an overly intense togetherness which alternated with some fairly intense emotional cutoffs. I started out, as most of us would, by focusing directly on the relationship with my mother and the one with my daughter. I soon discovered this wasn't something that could be turned around in mere weeks or months. Then eventually, learning from Murray Bowen that a two person relationship is "too small an arena" for solid change, I spread my attention out further into the family. I worked, ever so slowly, to change things with both my father and mother, with my brother and his family, with aunts and uncles, eventually with my son and daughter and their spouses and kids. I look, now, at the way my daughter deals with me and with her own infant daughter—more calmly than ever I was able—and I have a fair indication there's been a positive change in the familiar old chain of emotional cutoffs between mothers and daughters.

That was, admittedly, a long, laborious process, and I know most people see such an effort as too strenuous and time-consuming to be useful in the day-to-day work with persons with AIDS. Yet, through this sort of individual effort, I think family people have gained much knowledge that could be useful to others in their work with AIDS patients.

Where extended family work, itself, is concerned, that can be broken down into more manageable units than we usually think— depending on the amount of time there is to work with. For example: extra-long phone conversations with my mother, when I knew she had only a short time to live; 8 years doing genealogy with my father, toward the end of his life; 14 days he and I spent together in London when he was 85.

I also learned that I could be more effective in illness-related crises if I used some of the same principles that worked for me with my own family. For one thing, if I could get sufficiently neutral in the face of everyone's distress, I could more effectively get out of their way and let them make the best use of coping skills already in their repertoire. For another, I found it worked better to be less problem-oriented in the face of serious illness in a family—dealing much less with intense "issues" and working primarily to help people deal respectfully with one another and their different viewpoints. I never sent people back to confront, or to get their anger or hurt feelings out into the open; rather, my goal was to loosen up the relationship system sufficiently so that they could see one another as "just people," trying as best they knew how to get through life.

There are other ways, of course, to address the problems of families. There are individual therapies. There's conventional family group therapy, when workable. There are support groups: for the HIV positive, for persons with AIDS, for their partners, for their parents. There are multiple family groups, and educational groups. Then, since many people don't do well in groups, often because their ethnic or racial backgrounds mitigate against discussing family issues with strangers, there are at least a few people experimenting with different ways of providing services to these harder-to-reach clients.

I know full well that many persons with AIDS feel hurt and depreciated by their families, and thus have no interest in renewing contact with them. Conversely, there are parents who write off their children out of disappointment, hurt, or fear. Those situations are real and need to be respected as such. But the fact remains that emotional cutoffs such as these are never comfortable for any of the parties, and they do not ease life either for patient or family. I've had enough experience with long-term cutoffs in my family to know that I'd always *try* to increase contact, if only very slightly. I'd start in small ways like sending photographs, clippings, or audiotapes, even if they were not answered or were returned unopened. Or I'd contact peripheral family members, and count on the fact that information would move about the family through them, even if I was never informed of it. I'd make a project of that—not really counting on anything to happen but sort of playing around with the situation to see if I could get it loosened up somewhat and not so terribly intense and angry.

Recently I talked with a client about this notion of "family as the unit of care," and how important that seemed to me. She's a particularly intelligent woman, with whom I get into fairly theoretical and philosophical discussions. She came in originally to talk about a long-term lesbian relationship that seemed in trouble, and after the original crisis had resolved itself we began to look more closely at her relationships with extended family, particularly with brothers and sisters. Since both their parents are dead, and much of the original motivation to see one another now is lost, it took a little effort for her to begin to work in that direction. But she quickly caught onto the idea that whatever she managed to accomplish there would eventually generalize to the relationship with her lover and to other areas of her life.

At some point I was speculating about possible benefits of extended family contact for persons with AIDS. She reacted, as so many people do, by asking whether I thought people *owed* it to their families to reconnect with them—or whether I thought they *owed* something to future generations, by way of example. When we reached that impasse, I struggled to hear the meaning of her words, coming as they did from some experience with the illness and death of important friends—and she struggled to hear the meaning of my words as well. Finally, she said,

> I think I have a way to talk about that. I thought at first when you mentioned family that you meant going back to open up old issues with parents—I couldn't hear the idea as being broader than that. But, if I consider family to mean whatever a person chooses it to mean, *and then some*, I can begin to see it as a resource in a new way. For example, I have some cousins who might conceivably be at risk, and I know I'd want to be told if they were to develop AIDS. I'd like, at least, to have the choice to offer my help. I learned a lot from the experience of taking care of my mother as she was dying of cancer, and I think I would have much to contribute to others in my family who needed that kind of help.

It is important, I believe, to learn to see families in a more ecological way, as the "unit of care," expanding our view of family to include all sorts of valuable people, and excluding no one who might be a resource (or who might be affected by an AIDS diagnosis). My client's view of family clearly includes friends — and friends of friends — and cousins. And from my vantage point, it would certainly include parents — and grandparents. Should we perhaps include neighbors? Church congregations? Even whole towns?

As professionals working with persons with AIDS, with families of the chronically or terminally ill, or with families in general, I believe that *our thinking makes a major difference* in either limiting or increasing the human resources a person who is ill will be able to use in that critically important space of time. The Groves Task Force challenges us to expand our perspectives — to involve family in our thinking, as we search for solutions to the problems AIDS presents. This book can't do our thinking for us, but it does attempt to get us started.

G. Mary Bourne, ACSW
President and Director of Training
Minnesota Institute of Family Dynamics
Minneapolis, MN

Introduction

Eleanor D. Macklin, PhD

Sometimes in life there are projects which one feels called to do. For many of us who participated in this book, this was such an occasion. Once sensitized to the extremity of the AIDS (Acquired Immune Deficiency Syndrome) epidemic and to its potential for upending the lives of those whom it touches, persons in a position to make a difference will find it hard to look the other way.

THE STORY BEHIND THE BOOK

The history of this book and of the efforts of those responsible for its existence is, in many ways, a microcosm of what has happened to numerous other professionals in the human service field. It was Fall, 1985, when I first realized that AIDS was a topic about which I should be concerned. I was attending the annual meeting of the American Association for Marriage and Family Therapy in New York City, sitting with a friend knowledgeable about the cutting edge in medical research. In glancing at the program, he said, with concern, "There is not one paper being given on the topic of AIDS. You must do something about that." "But, I know nothing about AIDS," I replied. "It's not really my thing." "Well, then," he answered, "that will have to change." And, as it has turned out, he was right.

My logical first step was to submit a proposal to do a workshop on AIDS at the next meeting of the Groves Conference on Marriage

Eleanor D. Macklin is Associate Professor and Director of the Marriage and Family Therapy Program, College for Human Development, Syracuse University, Syracuse, NY 13244-1250.

1

and the Family. Groves Conference is a small interdisciplinary organization of scholars and professionals which meets annually for 5 days to discuss, in an atmosphere of thoughtful debate, the most pressing issues affecting the well-being of families and their members. It seemed a perfect forum to achieve the dialogue and leadership necessary if significant change was to occur. I felt considerable apprehension about the task I had undertaken. But so it has often been in this epidemic — many have had to act with little information and little time for preparation.

In the months before that July, 1986, meeting, I read everything I could get my hands on about AIDS, talked to any and all of my informed associates, and readied myself to share what I had learned. It was not an easy job. Every fact raised another question and every question took me deeper into areas I only vaguely understood — epidemiology, virology, the Gay community. But I was motivated. The more I read, the more aware I became of the urgency of the issues and of the fact that the human service community and, in particular, the family professionals were, with rare exception, totally oblivious to the crisis at their doorstep.

Only about 6 persons came to that workshop in Summer, 1986. But those of us who were there were united in concern. We went back to the general meeting and with some passion told the assemblage what we were learning. Sparks were ignited and the decision was made to establish an AIDS Task Force to explore ways to alert and to mobilize the professional community.

From there the movement grew steadily. An initial steering committee (Bruce Carter, Richard Needle, Jim Ramey, and myself) presented an open forum on AIDS at the November, 1986, annual meeting of the National Council on Family Relations (NCFR) in Dearborn. Attendance was modest, but better than it had been in July. A circle of maybe 25 persons listened and responded. A motion was made to the NCFR Board of Directors, requesting the formation of a NCFR AIDS Task Force. People were beginning to hear the message.

By April, 1987, when the Groves Conference met for their next annual meeting, the Groves Conference AIDS Task Force had grown to 45 persons (see membership listing at end of this volume). With the vision and persuasion of Mary Bourne, President and Director of Training, Minnesota Institute of Family Dynamics, monies were obtained from a private donor to pay the necessary expenses to bring these persons for 5 days to San Antonio to consider the issues which the AIDS epidemic raises for families and family professionals. They were a varied, talented, prestigious group, representing family scientists, AIDS specialists, and senior staff of many related professional organizations, including the Ackerman Institute for Family Therapy; American Association for Marriage and Family Therapy; American Association of Sex Educators, Counselors, and Therapists; Family Service America; The Hastings Center; The Kinsey Institute; Masters and Johnson Institute; National Council on Family Relations; National Hospice Organization; Planned Parenthood Federation of America; Sex Information and Education Council of the U.S.; and Society for the Scientific Study of Sex.

The 45 members of the Task Force were divided into 5 panels (Epidemiology and Public Health, Education and Prevention, Human Services and Treatment, Societal Implications, and Public Policy) and directed to consider the probable impact of the AIDS epidemic on individuals, families, and communities, and to delineate the implications for professionals, organizations, and public policy. They worked long and hard, talked into the night, and struggled with controversy. The essential principles, concerns, and realities enunciated during those discussions and developed over the ensuing months form the body of this volume.

This book is written primarily for professionals and policymakers who seek (a) to understand the realities of the AIDS epidemic and the problems which infection by the Human Immunodeficiency Virus (HIV, the virus responsible for AIDS) poses for individuals and their loved ones, and (b) to establish policies and procedures which may be useful in helping families and communities deal constructively with this epidemic. Being at risk for HIV infection, testing seropositive for HIV, or being diagnosed as having AIDS or ARC (AIDS-Related Complex) creates serious crises for individuals, their present and potential partners, their families and friends, and the human service workers and agencies who will be called upon for care and support. The complexity of the issues, the plethora of rapidly expanding knowledge, the fears and stigma often associated with AIDS, and the need for rational compassionate response make this epidemic a special challenge for the helping professional.

In the years since 1985 the professional community has made significant efforts to meet this challenge. Many human service and related professional organizations have established AIDS task forces and have made efforts to educate their membership (e.g., American Anthropological Association; American Association for Counseling and Development; American Association for Sex Educators, Counselors, and Therapists; American Family Therapy Association; American Orthopsychiatric Association; American Psychological Association; American Sociological Association; Family Service America; National Association of Social Workers; and Society for the Scientific Study of Sex). A number of significant professional reports have been released (e.g., Buckingham, 1988; Dalton & Burris, 1987; Griggs, 1986; The Institute of Medicine, National Academy of Sciences, 1986, 1988; *New England Journal of Public Policy*, 1988).

During the annual meeting of NCFR, November, 1987, in Atlanta, Georgia, the National Coalition on AIDS and Families was organized in order to extend the work of the Groves Conference Task Force (see end of this volume for Coalition goal statement and members of the steering committee). The Coalition is an association of professionals concerned about and sensitive to the issues which the HIV epidemic raises for families and their members and committed to working to achieve a humane and informed approach to this epidemic. Its goals are to help policymakers and human service professionals appreciate the implications of the HIV epidemic for families, both biological and functional, and to encourage the consideration of the family system in all educational efforts, service delivery, and policy development.

THE IMPACT OF THE HIV EPIDEMIC ON FAMILIES

The HIV epidemic has spread rapidly, and the numbers of infected persons appear to increase geometrically. The first AIDS-related cases were reported by the Centers for Disease Control on June 5, 1981. By September 3, 1982, 593 confirmed cases had been identified within the U.S., and 243 of these were already dead (McLaughlin, 1988). As of January 30, 1989, over 83,000 persons in the U.S had been diagnosed with AIDS, 56% of whom had already died (Centers for Disease Control, 1989). Another 1 to 1.5 million persons in the U.S. are estimated to be HIV-infected and, hence, contagious, and most of these eventually will develop severe HIV-related infections (Watkins et al., 1988). It is likely that as many as 10 million are infected worldwide, with more than 3 million infected in Africa. Recent estimates suggest that, by 1992, almost 500,000 persons in the U.S. will have died or progressed to the later stages of the disease (Watkins et al., 1988), and many thousands more will be asymptomatic HIV-infected. Although AIDS probably will increase predominantly in the low-income sections of large urban areas, it is clear that many persons in our society will be related to or care about someone who is infected with HIV.

To date, attention has been focussed primarily on those individuals diagnosed with ARC or AIDS, and on ways of providing for their care and treatment. Only slowly have we come to accept the need to focus on the full course of HIV infection and to realize that AIDS is only the end of the disease process. And only slowly have we come to recognize that for every infected individual there are numerous family members and loved ones—partners and spouses, parents and children, siblings and grandparents, friends and caregivers—whose lives also are affected significantly and who also need care and support.

There are many characteristics of the HIV epidemic which contribute to its significant impact on the entire family system. HIV infection is a potentially lethal disease. The average time between infection and the development of significant clinical symptoms is 7 to 8 years (Watkins et al., 1988). Although approximately 10% live at least 5 more years, the majority die within 2 to 3 years of being diagnosed with AIDS. Hence, to be seropositive or to be diagnosed as having an HIV-related infection means that the life of the individual will be severely shortened—a reality not easily accepted, especially when that individual is likely to be in the prime of life. Moreover, the behaviors which have been primarily responsible for the transmission of HIV (i.e., homosexual intercourse and intravenous drug use) are socially disapproved of by many, and a diagnosis of HIV infection often means disclosure to family and friends of behaviors which they may not accept.

Because the virus can be transmitted via semen and vaginal secretions, the sexual lives of individuals and their partners are directly and severely affected. Because a woman who is infected may transmit the virus to her child during pregnancy or at birth, increasing numbers of babies are being born HIV-positive and women at risk for infection face difficult decisions about childbearing. Four to five percent of pregnant women in some inner-city clinics currently are infected and one in every 61 babies born in New York City in mid-1988 was seropositive at birth (Watkins et al., 1988). Because the majority of women who are infected are asymptomatic and, hence, unaware of their infection, infants born with HIV infection are usually the first member of the family to be diagnosed. With parents unable to care for them, many of these infants will need foster care if they are to leave the hospital setting (for problems related to HIV-infected children, see Cooper, 1988; Klug, 1986; Urwin, 1988). Because the screening of blood for HIV was not possible until Spring, 1985, many persons who were given blood transfusions or blood products between 1977 and 1985 received infected blood. Hence, it is estimated that approximately 12,000 hemophiliacs are HIV-infected and, to date, 5% to 20% of their spouses also have become infected (Watkins et al., 1988).

There are many other implications of HIV infection for family life. Families play a key role in the education of their members regarding the transmission of HIV and in the development of informed and compassionate attitudes toward persons infected with HIV. HIV-infected persons require a wide variety of increasing medical care over the course of their illness, primarily to contend with the many opportunistic infections which their damaged immune systems cannot combat, and much of this care will occur at home. The discrimination against HIV-infected persons often extends to discrimination against their families and frequently exists even within these families, with members fearful of contamination by association with one another. Professionals who provide pre- and post-HIV test counseling must be sensitive to the complex emotional implications of either positive *or* negative test results for the individual and his/her relationships. Professionals who learn of their client's serostatus must struggle with the ethical issues surrounding confidentiality when these clients refuse to share this information with their sexual partners (e.g., see Gray & Harding, 1988).

It is impossible to overemphasize the profound emotional and economic costs of HIV infection for the entire family unit. The following are real-life examples of how the epidemic affects families and other such intimate relationships (Macklin, 1988):

- The grandmother in the inner-city slum with three grandchildren to care for, two of whom are sick with AIDS, who has already lost a daughter to AIDS due to infection by her drug-using boyfriend.
- The mother who learns of her own HIV infection only after her second child is born with AIDS, who fears the father's wrath for having infected his only son, and who worries about who will care for her children when she is gone.
- The gay couple whose parents urge the well partner to leave in order to protect himself (would they suggest that of a heterosexual married couple?), who fear that any physical closeness will infect the other, who struggle with whether the non-ill partner should be tested to see if he is already infected and with how they will handle a positive or negative outcome of such testing.
- The mother, whose son had died of AIDS, who asks for an HIV antibody test so that she can prove to her daughter that she is safe to visit her grandchildren.
- The bisexual man who has not told his wife of his lifestyle and who, when he learns that he is seropositive, agonizes over whether he has infected her, fears telling her, fears suggesting the use of a condom because she will suspect, fears not using a condom, thinks of her desire to become pregnant, and eventually distances himself in order to avoid dealing with the emotional pain.
- The mother who calls a Big Brother/Big Sister Program and asks for help for her two sons whose father has recently died from AIDS and who is told that the agency will not be able to help her.

- The wife whose husband has had an affair and who has convinced herself that he has given her AIDS even though she has received two negative test results.
- The mother who learns simultaneously that she is seropositive and pregnant for the first time and anguishes over whether or not to have an abortion.
- The student who finds a notice in a lover's desk that he has tested positive and then fears telling him, because he will know that she was snooping, and fears telling her regular boyfriend because he will be so angry at her.
- The parent who worries about the risk of HIV infection for his/her teenage offspring but does not know how to talk to them in a way which will affect their behavior.

Little has been published to date on the effect of HIV infection on the family or on the effect of fear of infection on intimate relationships in general. The exceptions to this include: (a) personal and clinical accounts of the experience of living with a loved one with AIDS (e.g., Burns, 1988; Carl, 1986; Helmquist, 1984; Peabody, 1986; Schreiber, 1988); (b) some excellent handbooks for family members and friends of infected persons (e.g., Martelli, Peltz, & Messina, 1987; Moffatt, 1986); and (c) the pioneering efforts of the Ackerman Institute for Family Therapy (see Mohr, Patten, Kaplan, & Gilbert, 1988; Walker, G., 1987, 1988; Walker, L., 1987) and Tiblier (1987). There are, as yet, no data on the family roles of persons with AIDS or on the number of family members typically infected in any given household. With few exceptions (e.g., Cleveland, Walters, Skeen, & Robinson, 1988; McMillan, 1988), there has been little systematic research on the reactions or potential reactions of families to an infected member. The interface between the HIV epidemic and human relationships is a research area crying for attention (see chapters by Carter and Needle & Leach in this volume for further discussion of research needs). Some significant projects with a family focus were funded in 1988 and will serve as models for others (e.g., Training for Health-Care Providers to Address Acquired Immune Deficiency Syndrome [AIDS], Division of Family Programs, Department of Psychiatry, University of Rochester Medical School; Twin Cities' IV-Drug/AIDS Research and Demonstration Project, Department of Family Social Science, University of Minnesota; Natural History of HIV Infection in the Family System, Walter Reed Army Medical Center, Washington, DC).

HIV affects not only the person who contracts the disease but everyone who lives with and cares about that individual. Family members and lovers must deal with denial, fear, anger, guilt, ambivalence, confusion, uncertainty, anguish, despair, secrecy, discrimination, change in relationship and in future goals, lack of access to services, high medical costs, and potential loss of income and housing. The impact of the crisis, and of the family system's response to that crisis, will extend far beyond the death of the infected family member. Low-income minority families, already overstressed and disproportionately infected, will bear a special burden.

Policymakers and human service professionals must remember that HIV infection exists within a significant social/emotional context and must seek ways to support the family system of which the infected person is a part. To do otherwise is to waste the potential resources of that family unit and to miss the opportunity for the healing and growth of relationships which can occur when the crisis is handled constructively and compassionately.

Appreciation for help in the development of this volume is extended to the Board of Directors of Groves Conference on Marriage and the Family and, in particular, to Pauline Boss, Roger Rubin, Virginia Sibbison, and Marvin Sussman for their leadership and support; to the members of the Groves Conference AIDS Task Force and, in particular, to the chairpersons of the subpanels of the Task Force—Elaine Anderson, Bruce Carter, Jeri Hepworth, Richard Needle, and Kay Tiblier—for their dedication, energy, perseverance, and wisdom; to Sandra Caron, Conference Coordinator for the Task Force and right-hand person throughout the project; to Jim Ramey for his support at the beginning when the task appeared overwhelming; to Mary Bourne for her patience and ability to convince others to share her faith in the significance of our project; to John G. Kellogg for his extensive financial contributions to the functioning of the Task Force; to Ralph Burant of Family Service America for providing helpful commentary on early drafts of the attached papers; to Sandra Davis for her thoughtful copyediting;

and to Dianne Miller for her expert secretarial skills and long hours. This project has been a labor born of conviction and concern. It serves as one more example of the kind of dedication which has been stimulated so often by the HIV crisis.

REFERENCES

Buckingham, S. (Ed.). (1988). AIDS: A special issue of *Social Casework*, *69*(6), 324-408.

Burns, I. (1988). We were there. *New England Journal of Public Policy*, *4*(1), 307-314.

Carl, D. (1986). Acquired Immune Deficiency Syndrome: A preliminary examination of the effects on gay couples and coupling. *Journal of Marital and Family Therapy*, *12*(3), 241-247.

Centers for Disease Control. (1989, January 30). *AIDS Weekly Surveillance Report*. Atlanta, GA: CDC.

Cleveland, P. H., Walters, L. H., Skeen, P., & Robinson, B. E. (1988). If your child had AIDS . . . Responses of parents with homosexual children. *Family Relations*, *37*, 150-153.

Cooper, E. R. (1988). AIDS in children: An overview of the medical, epidemiological, and public health problems. *New England Journal of Public Policy*, *4*(1), 121-133.

Dalton, H. L., & Burris, S. (Eds.). (1987). *AIDS and the law*. New Haven, CT: Yale University Press.

Gray, L. A., & Harding, A. K. (1988). Confidentiality limits with clients who have the AIDS virus. *Journal of Counseling and Development*, *66*, 219-223.

Griggs, J. (Ed.). (1986). *AIDS: Public policy dimensions*. New York: United Hospital Fund of New York.

Helmquist, M. (1984). *The family guide to AIDS: Responding with your heart*. San Francisco: San Francisco AIDS Foundation.

Institute of Medicine, National Academy of Sciences. (1986). *Confronting AIDS: Directions for public health, health care, and research*. Washington, DC: National Academy Press.

Institute of Medicine, National Academy of Sciences. (1988). *Confronting AIDS: Update 1988*. Washington, DC: National Academy Press.

Klug, R. (1986). Children with AIDS. *American Journal of Nursing*, *86*, 1126-1132.

Macklin, E. D. (1988). AIDS: Implications for families. *Family Relations*, *37*, 141-149.

McLaughlin, L. (1988). AIDS: An overview. *New England Journal of Public Policy*, *4*(1), 15-35.

McMillan, C. (1988, September). Families in Crisis: Coping with AIDS. *Focus: A Guide to AIDS Research*, *3*(10), 1-3.

Martelli, L. J., Peltz, F. D. P., & Messina, W. (1987). *When someone you know has AIDS: A practical guide*. New York: Crown Publishers.

Moffatt, B. C. (1986). *When someone you love has AIDS: A book of hope for family and friends*. New York: Penguin Books.

Mohr, R., Patten, J., Kaplan, L. S., & Gilbert, J. (1988). AIDS and family therapy. *The Family Therapy Networker, 12*(1), 33-43, 81.

New England Journal of Public Policy. (1988, Winter/Spring), *4*(1), 525 pp. (Special issue on AIDS.)

Peabody, B. (1986). *The screaming room: A mother's journal of her son's struggle with AIDS*. San Diego: Oak Tree Publications.

Schreiber, R. (1988). Accounts of an illness: Extracts. *New England Journal of Public Policy, 4*(1), 403-410.

Tiblier, K. (1987). Intervening with families with young adults with AIDS. In M. Wright and M. L. Leahey (Eds.), *Families and life-threatening illness*. St. Louis: Springhouse.

Urwin, C. A. (1988). AIDS in children: A family concern. *Family Relations, 37*, 154-159.

Walker, G. (1987, April/June). AIDS and family therapy. *Family Therapy Today, 2*(4,6).

Walker, G. (1988). An AIDS journal. *The Family Therapy Networker, 12*(1), 22-32, 76-79.

Walker, L. A. (1987, June 21). What comforts AIDS families. *New York Times Magazine*, pp. 16-22, 63, 78.

Watkins, J. D. et al. (1988). *Report of the Presidential Commission on the Human Immunodeficiency Virus Epidemic*. (Write: Presidential Commission, 655 15th St., Suite 901, Washington, D.C. 20005).

Chapter 1

The Human Immunodeficiency Virus (HIV) Epidemic: Epidemiological Implications for Family Professionals

Richard H. Needle, PhD, MPH
Susan Leach, RN, MN
Robin P. Graham-Tomasi, MPH

Home is the place where, when you have to go there, they have to take you in.

Robert Frost

INTRODUCTION

By January 30, 1989, almost 8 years after the first cases of what is now known as AIDS (Acquired Immunodeficiency Syndrome) were reported to the Centers for Disease Control, hereafter referred to as CDC, 83,592 persons in the U.S. had been diagnosed with

Richard H. Needle is affiliated with the Department of Family Social Science and School of Public Health and Susan Leach is affiliated with the Department of Family Social Science, 290 McNeal Hall, University of Minnesota, St. Paul, MN 55108. Robin P. Graham-Tomasi is affiliated with the Department of Family Social Science, University of Minnesota, and the Department of Health Behavior and Health Education, University of Michigan, M20 Washington Heights, Ann Arbor, MI 48109-2029.

This paper was supported in part by the Agricultural Experiment Station of the University of Minnesota. The authors would like to acknowledge the assistance of Dr. Marian P. Needle and Ms. Joan Kukowski.

13

AIDS, and over 48,582 men, women, and children had died from AIDS (CDC, 1989). AIDS is a syndrome of diseases resulting from a deterioration of an individual's immune system caused by infection by the human immunodeficiency virus (HIV). For this reason, HIV-infected persons, compared to individuals with normal immune systems, are susceptible to many infections (Institute of Medicine, 1986). It is these opportunistic infections[1] and certain types of cancer (e.g., Kaposi's sarcoma) that take advantage of the body's lowered immune system and eventually cause death. By early 1988, AIDS cases had been reported in 136 of 173 reporting countries or territories, resulting, as of March 1988, in a total of 84,256 reported cases of AIDS worldwide (CDC, 1988a).

Considerable progress has been made since 1981 in understanding the disease syndrome, the determinants and distribution of the disease pattern in population groups, the evolving biology of AIDS, the clinical manifestations accompanying the progression of this infection, and means to prevent and control the spread of this epidemic. Three distinct global epidemiological patterns of HIV infection have been reported, differing in terms of when the virus was introduced and began to spread and the groups most affected. The modes of transmission are the same (sexual contact with infected persons, exposure to contaminated blood, and from an infected mother to her child during pregnancy or at birth), although the proportion of cases resulting from these various modes, and the social, economic, and political impact, vary considerably around the world (Piot et al., 1988). In Africa, the Caribbean, and some areas in South America, the virus was introduced or began to spread extensively in the early to late 1970s, and the main population group affected has been heterosexuals. For North America, Western Europe, and several other countries in South America, Australia, and New Zealand, HIV was introduced in the mid-1970s to the early '80s, and the major groups affected have been homosexual/bisexual men and intravenous drug users. More recently, the virus has begun to affect heterosexual and homosexual people in countries in Asia, the Pacific region, the Middle East, and Eastern Europe.

The magnitude of this epidemic and estimates of the impact generally are based on reported cases of AIDS and associated fatality rates, which are underreported in the United States and seriously underreported in the world. A truer estimate of the potential impact also has to take into account those currently infected with HIV who have not yet been diagnosed with AIDS. It is estimated that 1 to 1.5 million Americans currently are infected with HIV (Watkins et al., 1988). Worldwide, it is estimated that there are between 5 and 10 million HIV-infected people (Mann, 1988). Estimates of the percentages of currently HIV-infected persons who eventually will develop AIDS increase annually. Although the impact of this epidemic, from an epidemiological perspective, is often represented in terms of numbers of infected persons, the number of persons affected is much greater. HIV affects not only the individuals who are infected, but also their predecessor families and families of succession, whether biological or not. The proportion of Americans who report knowing someone with AIDS has increased from 4% in October 1986, to 6% in October 1987, to 7% in 1988 (Dawson, Cynamon, & Fitti, 1988).

The purpose of this paper is to examine the epidemiology of HIV infection and AIDS. It is helpful to consider 3 interrelated but distinct phases of this global epidemic (Mann, 1988). First is the epidemic of HIV infection, which is followed by the AIDS epidemic. Last is the epidemic of economic, social, political, and cultural reactions to HIV infection and AIDS. The implications for families[2] of all 3 epidemics will be discussed in other papers in this volume. This paper is not intended to be an exhaustive review of AIDS from an epidemiological perspective. Outstanding papers on this topic are readily available (Allen & Curran, 1988; Curran et al., 1988; Francis & Chin, 1987; Guinan & Hardy, 1987; Jaffe et al., 1985; Pyun, Ochs, Duffort, & Wedgwood, 1987; Quinn, 1987; also see Institute of Medicine, National Academy of Sciences, 1988; Watkins et al., 1988). Rather, the present paper selectively interprets the epidemiology of HIV infection for nonmedical family practitioners who, in a continuing crisis, require information in order to work effectively with individuals and their family members.

AIDS EPIDEMIOLOGY

Population Groups at Risk for HIV Infection

In the middle of 1981, several outbreaks of Pneumocystis carinii pneumonia and Kaposi's sarcoma in previously healthy young male homosexuals were reported to the CDC (CDC, 1981a, 1981b). Prior to these reports, these diseases usually were diagnosed only in persons with recognized causes of immune system compromise, such as rare genetic diseases, immunosuppressive treatments for organ transplants, and cancer chemotherapy.

By the end of 1982, 738 cases of AIDS had been reported and additional groups were represented among these cases: IV drug users, hemophiliacs, transfusion recipients, female sexual partners of men at risk for AIDS, and infants born to infected mothers. These high-risk groups have not changed over the course of the epidemic and are similar all over the world, although the proportion of cases in these categories is changing over time. The numbers of AIDS cases to date in the U.S. as of January 30, 1989, by transmission categories, are reported in Table 1.

It is now evident that it is not group membership (such as race/ethnicity, gender, occupation, or socioeconomic status) that creates the risk for HIV infection, but rather (a) specific behavioral practices of individuals that make them vulnerable to HIV infection (e.g., unprotected sexual intercourse with an infected individual or drug users sharing contaminated needles); (b) receiving contaminated blood or blood products; or (c) an HIV-infected mother transmitting the infection to her child during pregnancy or delivery.

Geographical Distribution

The distribution of reported AIDS cases by geographic region has changed markedly. Initially, AIDS was reported in major urban centers, particularly New York City and San Francisco. Today, even though the majority of cases is still from those cities, the proportion of cases from the rest of the United States has increased substantially (CDC, 1989). By mid-1988 over 14,000 of the total 65,000 AIDS cases had been reported in the New York City standard metropolitan statistical area (SMSA). Other SMSAs of varying sizes with more than 1,000 cases were, in order of numbers of cases, San Francisco, Los Angeles, Houston, Washington, D.C., Newark, Chicago, Miami, Dallas, Philadelphia, and Atlanta (CDC, 1988b). By 1991, 80% of all pediatric AIDS cases will occur out-

Table 1

United States Adult/Adolescent AIDS Cases Reported to Centers for Disease Control (as of January 30, 1989)[a]

Transmission Categories	Males No.	Males %	Females No.	Females %	Total No.	Total %
Homosexual/Bisexual Males	51,581	68	–	–	51,581	62
IV Drug Users	12,929	17	3,743	52	16,672	20
Homosexual Males and IV Drug Users	6,013	8	–	–	6,013	7
Hemophilia/Coagulation Disorder	775	1	23	0	798	1
Heterosexual Cases	1,555	2	2,130	30	3,685	4
Transfusion, Blood/Components	1,319	2	762	11	2,081	2
Undetermined	2,223	3	539	7	2,762	3
Total of Adult/Adolescent	76,395	91	7,197	9	83,592	100

a As reported in AIDS Weekly Survelliance Report -- United States AIDS Program, Center for Infectious Diseases, Centers for Disease Control, January 30, 1989, Table A.

side of New York and San Francisco, the cities most greatly affected by AIDS to date (U.S. House of Representatives, 1988a).

The distribution of AIDS cases by selected risk factors varies
geographically. For example, whereas by mid-1988 63% of the total AIDS cases in the United States had been related to gay/bisexual
contact, only 58% of all AIDS cases in New York State had been
classified as homosexual/bisexual, compared to 92% of all cases in
California. New York and, to a greater extent, New Jersey report
higher percentages of AIDS cases among IV drug users. In 1988, in
New Jersey, 48% of all AIDS cases were IV drug users; in New
York, 33%; and in California, 2.5%. The geographic variation in
percentage of reported AIDS cases from blood or blood products
has varied from about 1.5% to 6% of total cases (Allen & Curran,
1988).

Racial and Ethnic Characteristics

This epidemic has had a disproportionate impact on minority populations, particularly the Black and Hispanic populations in our
country. As of early 1989, 27% of total adult cases were Black and
14% were Hispanic, although Blacks are 11.6% and Hispanics 6.5%
of the U.S. population (Curran et al., 1988; CDC, 1989). Of the total pediatric cases, 52% were Black and 23% were Hispanic (see
Table 2).

The disproportionately higher rates of AIDS among Blacks and
Hispanics reflect higher reported rates among Black and Hispanic
IV drug users, their sexual partners, and their infants (Curran et al.,
1988). In the adult population as of mid-1988, 50% of IV drug-use
AIDS cases were Black not Hispanic, 29% were Hispanic, and 19%
were White not Hispanic.[3] Cases of AIDS among Blacks and Hispanics also are reported in the other transmission categories.

Age Distribution

This epidemic has affected mostly young and middle-aged males
and females, though cases have been reported for infants, adolescents, and older individuals. Of all the reported cases of AIDS as of
early 1989, 46% had occurred in the 30-39 year-old age group, and
21% in each of those aged 20-29 and 40-49. As of January 30,

Table 2

Pediatric AIDS Cases[1] by Transmission Category and Racial-Ethnic Group (cumulative as of January 30, 1989)[2]

	White, Not Hispanic		Black, Not Hispanic		Hispanic		Other/ Unknown		TOTAL	
	Number	(%)	Number	(%)	Number	(%)	Number	(%)	Number	(%)
Hemphilia/Coagulation Disorder	61	(18)	10	(1)	11	(4)	2	(25)	84	(6)
Parent with/at risk of AIDS	166	(50)	648	(89)	260	(81)	4	(50)	1080	(78)
Transfusion, Blood/Components	98	(29)	39	(5)	36	(11)	2	(25)	175	(13)
Undetermined	10	(3)	31	(4)	13	(4)	-	-	54	(4)
TOTAL [% of all cases]	335	[24]	728	[52]	320	[23]	8	[1]	1393	[100]

1   Includes all patients under 13 years of age at time of diagnosis.
2   As reported in AIDS Weekly Survelliance Report -- United States AIDS Program, Center for Infectious Diseases, Centers for Disease Control, January 30, 1989, Table B.

1989, 1,393 cases of AIDS had been reported for children under 13 years of age at time of diagnosis (CDC, 1989).

MODES AND RATES OF TRANSMISSION
OF HIV INFECTION

Even before HIV was identified as the etiological (causative) agent in 1983-1984 (Barre-Sinoussi et al., 1983; Gallo et al., 1984), it was hypothesized that the infectious agent was transmitted sexually, through parenteral exposure (direct contact with the bloodstream) to infected blood and blood products, and from infected mother to child during pregnancy. Early analysis of the epidemiological data suggested that the modes of transmission for groups at risk for AIDS was similar to those for hepatitis B (Institute of Medicine, 1986).

Epidemiological data have confirmed that AIDS is a disease spread through (a) sexual contact with an infected person involving exchange of body fluids (semen, blood, vaginal secretions); (b) direct exposure to infected blood, primarily by sharing contaminated drug needles or by transfusion of HIV-contaminated blood or blood components; and (c) transmission from an infected mother to her infant before birth, at the time of delivery, or possibly through breast milk (Rogers, 1987). Sources of transmission and non-transmission are briefly discussed in this section.

Sexual Transmission

The most common mode of HIV transmission is sexual contact with an HIV-infected person. It is primarily transmitted through vaginal or anal intercourse, and it can be spread from male to female, female to male, and male to male. Female-to-female transmission, although extremely rare, has been reported (Curran et al., 1988). Sexual behaviors, not sexual orientation, increase/decrease the risk of acquiring HIV infection. Risk for HIV infection depends on a number of factors, such as the number of sexual partners, the probability that a sexual partner is HIV-infected, the type of sexual activity, the correct use of condoms, duration of infection in the partner, clinical status of the partner, and the presence of genital lesions in either partner (CDC, 1978b; Fineberg, 1988; Moss et al., 1987). HIV has been isolated from blood, semen, and cervical secretions, can be transmitted during heterosexual or homosexual intercourse, and can enter the body through the vagina, penis, or rectum (Koop, 1988). The risk of acquiring HIV infection from a single sexual encounter with an infected person remains unknown at this time (Friedland & Klein, 1987), yet infection can occur from a single sexual contact (Mann, 1988).

Homosexual transmission. Among gay or bisexual men, the most greatly affected group, sexual contact is the primary mode of transmission of HIV. As of January 30, 1989, gay and bisexual men accounted for 62% (N = 51,581) of the reported adult/adolescent cases without any other known risk factors (CDC, 1989). The percentage of AIDS cases in which the risk factor is homosexual contact has varied geographically from 92% in California to 58% in New York (Allen & Curran, 1988). Anal intercourse, specifically receptive anal intercourse without the use of condoms, has been demonstrated to be a major risk factor for HIV infection (Kingsley et al., 1987; Office of Technical Assistance, 1988). Seroprevalence (the number of HIV-infected individuals) among this group has ranged from 10% to 70% depending on geographical area (CDC, 1987b).

There is substantial evidence that gay and bisexual men have made many risk-reducing behavioral changes (Becker & Joseph, 1988; McKusick, Wiley, & Coates, 1985), thus reducing the probabilities of acquiring and transmitting HIV infection. Change has not been uniform within groups whose behaviors put them at risk of HIV infection, and greater behavior change has occurred in higher prevalence areas (OTA, 1988).

Heterosexual transmission. Since 1983, when the first evidence for heterosexual transmission was reported (CDC, 1983), there has been a steady increase in the number of persons with AIDS for whom the only risk factor was heterosexual contact with a person known to be HIV-infected or at risk for such infection. Heterosexual transmission can occur in heterosexual partners of HIV-seropositive IV drug users, female sex partners of HIV-infected bisexual men, sexual partners of infected hemophiliacs or persons infected through transfusion, clients of infected prostitutes, and the heterosexual partners of other infected individuals. The prevalence of HIV infection in heterosexual partners of persons with HIV infection varies from 0% to 60%, although, at the present time, it is not clear what accounts for these differences (CDC, 1987b). The rates of heterosexual spread are highest among partners of IV drug users having unprotected sexual intercourse over extended periods (Curran et al., 1988). As of July 11, 1988, 2,761 cases of heterosexual AIDS with no other known risk factor, accounting for 4% of the total cases, had been reported (CDC, 1988a). Heterosexual transmission is most likely the leading route of HIV infection worldwide (see Friedland & Klein, 1987, for a review).

Transmission Through Exposure to Blood or Blood Products

Transmission through sharing drug equipment. The risk of contracting and transmitting AIDS among drug users depends on sharing injection equipment; the number of people sharing needles, syringes, and other paraphernalia; and the number of times equipment is shared with persons who are HIV-infected. There is also recent concern that crack users are engaging in sexual activity for money, thus increasing the possibility of contracting HIV infection and other STDs.

As of January 30, 1989, intravenous drug users accounted for 20% (N = 16,672) of adult/adolescent AIDS cases (CDC, 1989). In addition, there were 6,013 cases of AIDS where 2 risk factors were present: male homosexual contact and IV drug use. There are about 1.1 to 1.3 million IV drug users in the U.S. Overall, between 70% and 90% of IV drug users are thought to share use of injection equipment, resulting in high risk for contracting and transmitting AIDS (Schuster, 1988). Needle-sharing practices and seroprevalence rates vary by city. In the New York City area, the seroprevalence rate has ranged from 50% to 65%; in areas other than the East Coast, the seroprevalence rate among IV drug users has been mainly below 5% (CDC, 1987b). (For a more thorough discussion of needle sharing among IV drug users, see Battjes and Pickens, 1988.)

Infected intravenous drug users are the major bridge for heterosexual and perinatal transmission of HIV. About 75% of IV drug users are males (OTA, 1988). Most male IV drug users are heterosexual (Drucker, 1986) and most have their primary sexual relationship with women who are not IV drug users (Des Jarlais et al., 1984). Moreover, 52% of all women diagnosed with AIDS are IV drug users (see Table 1), and 30% to 50% of female IV drug users have engaged in prostitution at some time in their drug-using histories (Drucker, 1986). Recent reports indicate an increase in risk-reduction behaviors among IV drug users, such as increased use of clean needles and/or the cleaning of needles and reduced needle-sharing (Becker & Joseph, 1988). However, at the Fourth International Conference on AIDS in 1988 it was reported (Des Jarlais, 1988) that a question remains whether IV drug users are also changing their sexual practices, using condoms or reducing the number of partners.

Transmission through blood transfusions and blood products. Early in the epidemic, it was demonstrated that the infectious agent, later to be named HIV, could be transmitted through infected blood or blood products from donors to transfusion recipients. Certain blood products, notably Factor VIII taken by hemophiliacs to prevent coagulation problems, could also be contaminated. To date, 2% of the adult/adolescent cases and 13% of the pediatric cases have occurred through blood transfusions and blood products (see Tables 1 and 2).

For hemophiliac men in the U.S., seroprevalence rates ranging from 33% to 92% and 14% to 52% have been reported among those diagnosed with Hemophilia A and Hemophilia B respectively (CDC, 1987a). As of June 1988, it was estimated that approximately 12,000 hemophiliacs were HIV-infected and that 5% to 20% of their spouses were also infected (see Watkins et al., 1988; also see CDC, 1987a for discussion of related research).

Following the discovery of the HIV virus in 1984, tests have been developed to detect antibodies to HIV. Blood, plasma, and blood products used by hemophiliacs currently are screened, substantially reducing the risks for transfusion-associated AIDS and HIV infection among hemophiliacs (Petricciani & Epstein, 1988).

Transmission through infected blood in health-care settings. Laboratory workers and health-care personnel who provide care to persons with HIV infection are considered to be at some risk because of their occupational exposure to infected blood, but the risk is low. Health-care workers who become HIV-infected, like persons in other occupations, do so through the primary modes of transmission: IV needle-sharing and sexual contact with infected persons. Three prospective studies (Gerberding, Bryant-LeBlanc, & Nelson, 1987; Henderson et al., 1986; Weiss et al., 1988) to assess the risk for U.S. health-care workers of acquiring HIV infection have reported a very low risk of developing HIV antibodies, even following needlestick injuries or through exposures to laboratory specimens or other body fluids from patients with HIV infection.

Perinatal Transmission

Perinatal transmission accounts nationwide for 78% of cases of HIV infection in prepubertal children less than 13 years old. Infants born to mothers with HIV infection may become HIV-infected in 3 ways: (a) passage of the virus to the unborn baby through the placenta, (b) exposure to infected maternal blood and vaginal fluids during labor and delivery, and (c) ingestion of breast milk containing the virus (Rogers, 1987). In 1988, it was estimated that in New York City, about 3% of women of reproductive age were infected with HIV (U.S. House of Representatives, 1988a). An HIV-infected mother will transmit the virus to her infant in 20% to 60% of pregnancies (Watkins et al., 1988).

Unsubstantiated Transmission Sources

Other suspected modes of transmission, such as casual contact, insect bites, kissing, saliva, sweat, and toilet seats have been shown *not* to transmit HIV infection. There is *no* evidence of household transmission. Studies involving over 400 family members of HIV-infected individuals have found no evidence of transmission to members of the household who were not sexually involved with the infected individual (Rogers, 1987). People living with persons with AIDS, sharing their bathrooms and eating utensils, and hugging and kissing them at frequent intervals have not developed AIDS as a result of household contact (Friedland et al., 1986).

EPIDEMIOLOGY: GENERATIONAL IMPLICATIONS

Although attention has begun to focus on children with HIV infection and their families, and on AIDS and teenagers (Koop, 1987a; U.S. House of Representatives, 1988b), the generational significance of this epidemic and the impact on families has long been an obvious, though neglected, concern. By examining the different age groups affected by HIV and separately for males and females, our perspective on the impact of this epidemic will be broadened.

Men

Since the beginning of this epidemic, males have been most greatly affected and, as of January 30, 1989, accounted for 91% (76,395) of the number of reported AIDS cases in adults/adolescents (CDC, 1989). Most male cases of AIDS have been gay/bisexual men (68%), followed by heterosexual male IV drug users (17%) (CDC, 1989). In addition, 8% of male AIDS cases have had 2 risk factors: homosexuality and IV drug use. This epidemic has affected mostly young and middle-aged males, in their procreative and economically productive years. HIV-infected men are sons, spouses, lovers, fathers, and brothers. Their illness will affect many people who rely on them and care about them, and the reaction of these others will affect, in turn, their own lives.

Women

As of January 30, 1989, women constituted 9% (N = 7,197) of all AIDS cases (CDC, 1989). Of all women with AIDS, 52% were IV drug users and 30% contracted HIV infection heterosexually. Women with HIV/AIDS are the major source of infection for infants (Guinan & Hardy, 1987).

The number of women with AIDS has increased tremendously, from 51 cases in 1982 (CDC, 1983) to over 7,000 cases by early 1989 (CDC, 1989). Cases are expected to increase 600% to over

20,000 by the end of 1991 (U.S. House of Representatives, 1988a). The percentage of women with AIDS who have been infected via heterosexual contact has more than doubled from 14% in 1982 (Guinan & Hardy, 1987) to 30% in early 1989 (CDC, 1989). It may be easier for heterosexual women to acquire HIV infection than heterosexual men because a greater proportion of men are infected and the virus may be more efficiently transmitted from men to women (Guinan & Hardy, 1987).

Of women with AIDS, a disproportionate number are found in minority groups: in mid-1988, 51% were Black, 20% were Hispanic, and 28% were White (Watkins et al., 1988). In New York City alone, approximately 50,000 women of reproductive age are infected with HIV (U.S. House of Representatives, 1988a). It is estimated that there are 200,000 asymptomatic female carriers of the virus.

Over 80% of women with AIDS are between the ages of 13 and 39, the peak childbearing ages (Guinan & Hardy, 1987). Both symptomatic and asymptomatic women can transmit HIV to their infants. HIV-infected babies often are born to women who did not know they were HIV-positive or that their partners were in a risk group, and it was the infected infant who established the mother's diagnosis. Epidemiological data (Wofsy, 1987) suggest that women with AIDS have shorter survival times than men. This means that many mothers of HIV-infected newborn children will be ill, or become ill, and die soon after the birth of their child. Women with HIV infections are not only mothers to current and future generations, but daughters, spouses, lovers, and sisters who are in their economically productive years.

Children

Pediatric AIDS was recognized early in the epidemic, and, as of January 30, 1989, the number of reported cases had risen rapidly to a total of 1,393 cases under 13 years of age at time of diagnosis (see Table 2). For each case of AIDS in children, it is estimated that there are 3 to 5 times as many children with AIDS-related illnesses (U.S. House of Representatives, 1988a). It is estimated that, by 1991, there will be 10,000 to 20,000 symptomatic HIV-infected children in the U.S. (Watkins et al., 1988). As of January 1989, perinatal transmission accounted nationwide for 78% of all cases of HIV infection in prepubertal children less than 13 years of age. Because a positive antibody test in a newborn may be due to the presence of maternal antibodies, asymptomatic newborns may not be accurately diagnosed for 10 to 18 months (Watkins et al., 1988).

Pediatric HIV infection is characterized by a broad spectrum of disease, is associated with a high mortality rate, and has important differences from adult AIDS. Symptoms in infants include fever, rashes, diarrhea, small size, respiratory disease such as pneumonia, and enlargement of liver and spleen (Klug, 1986). In young children, even common childhood infections may be extremely serious due to their depressed immune systems. In infants and children, AIDS typically is characterized by serious bacterial infections and the failure to thrive. Survival rates are low; of all children diagnosed with AIDS before 1984, 75%-80% are dead (U.S. House of Representatives, 1988a).

Three-quarters of all children with AIDS are Black or Hispanic (see Table 2). Somewhat over 50% of all pediatric AIDS cases are among Blacks, though Black children represent only 15% of the total U.S. child population. Although 10% of the child population is Hispanic, as of early 1989 almost one-quarter of the cases of childhood AIDS were found in the Hispanic population. Twenty-four percent of the pediatric AIDS cases were found among White children, although 75% of the child population is White (U.S. House of Representatives, 1988a).

The child often is the first member of the family identified as infected. Testing of parents and siblings is then immediately indicated, and it is not unusual for both parents and one or more siblings to be HIV-positive. Therefore, the parents are confronted suddenly with issues regarding their own health status as well as that of the child. The number of families with more than one HIV-positive member is unknown (Boland, 1987).

The majority of HIV-infected children come from homes where one or both parents have a history of drug use, and the majority of families of pediatric AIDS are headed by a single parent, usually the mother (Boland, 1987). These families have multiple needs and will have to rely on community resources, such as health and human service agencies and foster care.

Adolescents

Although AIDS cases among 13-19 year-olds at time of diagnosis have been relatively few (342 as of January 30, 1989), cases among this age group increased by 54% over a ten-month period in 1987 (U.S. House of Representatives, 1988b). Behaviors such as high rates of sexual activity, low rates of condom usage, high rates of sexually-transmitted diseases, and use of drugs place adolescents at high risk. Because the time between infection with HIV and onset may be several years, some proportion of those in their 20s who have been diagnosed with AIDS probably became infected as teenagers (Koop, 1987b), an epidemiological fact that is causing great concern for professionals.

Modes of transmission of HIV infection in adolescents are similar to those for adults. Principally, they have become infected through receiving infected blood, through sexual activity with an infected partner, or through using contaminated needles. About 2.5 million teenagers experience sexually-transmitted diseases each year (U.S. House of Representatives, 1988a).

Use of drugs is widely prevalent in the adolescent population. Data from several sources indicate that use of illicit drugs by adolescents has the potential to increase the risk for HIV infection. In 1985 (the most recent data from the National Institute on Drug Abuse sponsored household survey), 5.2% of youth ages 12 to 17 reported having ever used cocaine (National Institute on Drug Abuse, 1986). Although the routes of administration of this drug vary, some adolescents are using this substance intravenously. Episodes of cocaine emergency room visits have increased recently in the 12- to 17-year-old age group, although drug emergencies, as well as prevalence, is highest in the young adult age group (NIDA, 1987). The epidemic of crack use has serious implications for youth because drug use and sexual activity often occur together. Use of heroin in the adolescent population is not highly prevalent. A number of cases of AIDS among adolescents have occurred among hemophiliacs. The impact of HIV infection on adolescents will be most profound for minority youth (U.S. House of Representatives, 1988b).

NATURAL HISTORY OF HIV INFECTION

The natural history of the disease and clinical manifestations of HIV infection range from asymptomatic (complete absence of symptoms) to mild AIDS-related conditions to severe conditions indicative of AIDS (Institute of Medicine, 1986; Landesman, Ginzburg, & Weiss, 1985; Melbye, 1986). Infection begins when HIV enters the bloodstream and stimulates the immune system to develop antibodies. The interval between HIV infection and the development of antibodies (or seroconversion) and the interval between infection with HIV and the first symptoms of AIDS (i.e., incubation period) vary from individual to individual. The usual time between infection by the virus and seroconversion has been estimated to be 6 to 8 weeks (Melbye, 1986).

It is the HIV antibodies, rather than the HIV virus itself, which are detected by the current blood tests. The tests for detecting HIV antibodies have proven to be very sensitive and specific (Francis & Chin, 1987). Two tests, the ELISA (enzyme-linked immunosorbent assay) and the more complicated Western Blot, are often performed in sequence to improve reliability (Miike, 1987). The ELISA is the most widely used HIV test because of its low cost, standardized procedure, and high reproducibility (Schwartz, Dans, & Kinosian, 1988). A current study by Wolensky (1988) suggests that the virus can remain hidden within the human body for more than 3 years before conventional tests are able to detect it. Several new tests for detecting evidence of HIV infection that screen for the virus, rather than the antibodies, are being developed.

Following initial infection and seroconversion, most persons with HIV infection remain asymptomatic for a period of time. Therefore, many people remain unaware that they are infected, yet they are capable of transmitting the virus to others. As more data have become available and more scientific investigations occur, estimates of the incubation period lengthen. The mean incubation period for homosexual men is estimated to be 7.8 years (Lui, Darrow, & Rutherford, 1988) and for adults developing transfusion-associated AIDS is 8.2 years. In children, the mean incubation period is considerably less.

When the virus has caused sufficient damage to the immune system, clinical symptoms appear. The majority of conditions accompanying HIV infection represent the results of immunologic damage rather than the direct effects of HIV infection. Clinical symptoms may first include the following: extreme fatigue, fever, diarrhea, weight loss, night sweats, swollen lymph nodes, and shortness of breath. Repeated infections and illnesses may drain the person's strength and result in life-threatening conditions. Because of progressive damage to the immune system, individuals may develop certain infections which seldom would cause disease in persons with normal defense mechanisms. These opportunistic diseases, common in the HIV/AIDS epidemic, include Pneumocystis carinii pneumonia, Kaposi's sarcoma, toxoplasmosis, tuberculosis, thrush, and meningitis (Institute of Medicine, 1986). As of January 30, 1989, the majority of reported cases of AIDS (60%) and known deaths from AIDS (59%) have been related to Pneumocystis carinii pneumonia (CDC, 1989).

In addition to these physical symptoms, the virus can directly affect the brain, causing a neurological syndrome, AIDS dementia complex, characterized by abnormalities in thinking, behavior, and movement (Price et al., 1988). This may result in such problems as forgetfulness, poor concentration, unsteady walking, and loss of control of arms and legs, thus impeding the person's ability to function independently. With time, these problems may become more severe, resulting in weakness, loss of speech, and lack of interest in usual activities.

A recent study (Marzuk et al., 1988) demonstrates a substantially increased risk for suicide among males with AIDS. Men aged 20 to 59 years with a diagnosis of AIDS are approximately 36 times more likely to commit suicide than their counterparts who have not received a diagnosis of AIDS, and 66 times more likely to commit suicide than members of the general population. Psychological stressors related to withdrawal of family support and loss of friends or lovers (often to AIDS) may serve as precipitating factors of suicide in persons with AIDS.

In the past, it was estimated that perhaps 5%-10% of people infected with HIV would develop AIDS, but recent evidence from continuing studies indicate that those estimates are not accurate. Projections from prospective cohort studies of infected persons suggest that more than 30% of HIV-infected persons will have AIDS within 7 years after they are infected and another 40% or more will have other clinical illnesses associated with HIV infection (Hessol et al., 1987). Some believe that, in time, all HIV-infected people will develop AIDS (Watkins et al., 1988).

SOCIETAL AND RESEARCH IMPLICATIONS

This paper provides a descriptive report of the epidemiology of the Human Immunodeficiency Virus/AIDS epidemic. Over 83,000 cases of AIDS had been reported in the United States as of January 30, 1989. Unfortunately, new cases from the current HIV-infected population will continue to develop, with the total projected to reach about 270,000 by the end of 1991 (Public Health Reports, 1986). Some of this increase will reflect growing numbers of infected women of childbearing age and, as more women become infected and bear children, increasing numbers of HIV infection in children. By 1991, the cumulative number of pediatric AIDS cases will have increased to 3,000 (Koop, 1987a).

The arithmetic of this epidemic dramatizes the need to (a) educate every individual about the prevention of AIDS; (b) develop, test, and make available drug therapies to those already infected with HIV to prevent the progression of the disease; and (c) accelerate the development, testing, and availability of a safe vaccine. Methods to prevent transmission of HIV are well established (see chapter by Hepworth and Shernoff in this volume): avoiding sexual behaviors which allow contact with HIV-infected semen or vaginal secretions, taking precautions to avoid contact with HIV-infected blood, not sharing needles with persons who may be HIV-infected, and testing for seropositivity before becoming pregnant. In May 1988, and years overdue, the Surgeon General's brief publication, *Understanding AIDS* (Koop, 1988), was mailed to all households in the U.S. in order to alert citizens to the need for prevention. Prevention strategies are extremely important given the fact that no vaccines are currently available. There is also an urgent need for less expensive, more effective, and more readily available drugs for the treatment of HIV infection. The most promising drug, azidothymidine (AZT), is very expensive, has negative side effects, and is not available to all who might benefit.

The economic consequences of HIV infection and AIDS for the individual and family can be devastating. The costs of necessary hospital inpatient care, ambulatory physician care, hospital outpatient care, emergency room care, and prescription medicine are enormous. The mean lifetime cost of medical care for one AIDS patient is estimated to be about $80,000 (Bloom & Carliner, 1988). The economic burden of direct and indirect costs eventually will have to be shared among patients, their families, employers, employees, taxpayers, health care systems, and the government (Fox & Thomas, 1987/1988).

The social impact of AIDS is enormous. The social, psychological, and economic needs of persons with AIDS will be absorbed mainly by caregivers, primarily family and loved ones. Those directly affected are sons and daughters, fathers and mothers, spouses and partners, brothers and sisters, infants and children, adolescents, and adults of every age. Families will be asked to provide assistance for the adult son with AIDS-related dementia and the 4-year-old daughter with yet another case of pneumonia. The implications for future generations are profound, although yet to be examined in a systematic manner.

Key epidemiological questions about AIDS and HIV infection will continue to be investigated, along with intense efforts to understand more clearly the biology of AIDS. Hopefully, drugs for the treatment of HIV infection will be developed and made available to those in need, and an effective vaccine to prevent infection will be discovered, although researchers are not optimistic about a vaccine in the near future. Along with research in the basic and applied sciences, it is essential that social scientists focus attention on the impact of the epidemic on the family and on the role of the family in prevention and control of the spread of HIV infection.

More specifically, it seems important to determine the immediate, cumulative, and changing demands associated with the natural history of HIV infection and related diseases for various risk groups and their families. For example, the potential impact of care-giving responsibilities on family members' physical and psychological help and overall family functioning requires attention. The description and understanding of coping resources and strategies available to and adopted by families and index patients across the natural history of HIV infection needs study. Furthermore, the relationships between family and community material resources, family coping, and family functioning and the physical and psychological well-being of the index patient require elucidation. Finally, further investigation of the financial costs to families and communities associated with health care and social support services over the natural history of HIV infection is called for.

NOTES

1. Opportunistic infections, such as Pneumocystis carinii pneumonia, tuberculosis, and some herpes viral infections, are caused by microorganisms that would most likely not cause disease in a person with normal defense mechanisms (Institute of Medicine, 1986, p. 46).

2. The definition of family used in this paper is "a social unit composed of members who have mutual obligations to provide a broad range of emotional and material support" (Dean, Lin, & Ensel, 1981).

3. This is the racial/ethnic classification system used by the weekly surveillance reporting by the Centers for Disease Control.

REFERENCES

Allen, J. R., & Curran, J. W. (1988). Prevention of AIDS and HIV infection: Needs and priorities for epidemiologic research. *American Journal of Public Health, 78*, 381-386.

Barre-Sinoussi, F., Chermann, J., Rey, F., Nugeyre, M., Chamaret, S., Gruest, J., Dauquet, C., Axler-Blin, C., Vezinet-Brun, F., Ronzioux, C., Rozenbaum, C., & Montaigner, L. (1983). Isolation of a T-lymphotropic retrovirus from a patient at risk for Acquired Immune Deficiency Syndrome (AIDS). *Science, 220*, 868-891.

Battjes, R. J., & Pickens, R. W. (Eds.). (1988). *Needle sharing among intravenous drug abusers: National and international perspectives.* (NIDA Research Monograph 80). Rockville, MD: National Institute on Drug Abuse.

Becker, M. H., & Joseph, J. G. (1988). AIDS and behavioral change to reduce risk: A review. *American Journal of Public Health, 78*, 394-410.

Bloom, D. E., & Carliner, G. (1988). The economic impact of AIDS in the United States. *Science, 239*, 604-610.

Boland, M. G. (1987). Management of the child with HIV infection: Implications for service delivery. In B. Silverman & H. Waddell (Eds.), *Report of the Surgeon General's Workshop on Children with HIV Infection and Their Families* (pp. 41-43). Washington, DC: Public Health Service.

Centers for Disease Control. (1981a, June 5). Pneumocystis pneumonia—Los Angeles. *Morbidity and Mortality Weekly Report, 30*, 250-252.

Centers for Disease Control. (1981b, July 3). Kaposi's sarcoma and Pneumocystis pneumonia among homosexual men—New York City and California. *Morbidity and Mortality Weekly Report, 30*, 305-308.

Centers for Disease Control. (1983, January 7). Immunodeficiency among female sexual partners of males with Acquired Immunodeficiency Syndrome (AIDS)—New York. *Morbidity and Mortality Weekly Report, 31*, 697-698.

Centers for Disease Control. (1987a, September 11). HIV infection and pregnancies in sexual partners of HIV-seropositive hemophiliac men—United States. *Morbidity and Mortality Weekly Report, 36*, 593-595.

Centers for Disease Control. (1987b, December 18). Human Immunodeficiency Virus infection in the United States: A review of current knowledge. *Morbidity & Mortality Weekly Report, 36* (Suppl. No. 506), 1-48.

Centers for Disease Control (1988b, May 13). Update: Acquired Immunodeficiency Syndrome (AIDS)—Worldwide. *Morbidity and Mortality Weekly Report, 37*, 286-295.

Centers for Disease Control. (1988b, July 11). *AIDS Weekly Surveillance Report*, United States AIDS Program, Center for Infectious Diseases.

Centers for Disease Control (1989, January 30). *AIDS Weekly Surveillance Report*, United States AIDS Program, Center for Infectious Diseases.

Curran, J. W., Jaffe, H. W., Hardy, A. M., Morgan, W. M., Selik, R. M., & Dondero, T. J. (1988). Epidemiology of HIV infection and AIDS in the United States. *Science, 239*, 610-616.

Dawson, D. A., Cynamon, M., & Fitti, J. (1988). AIDS knowledge and attitudes for September 1987, Provisional data from the National Health Interview Survey. *Advance Data from Vital and Health Statistics*. No. 148. DHHS Pub. No. (PHS) 88-1250. Hyattsville, MD: Public Health Service.

Dean, A., Lin, N., & Ensel, W. M. (1981). The epidemiological significance of social support systems in depression. In R. G. Simmons (Ed.), *Research in community mental health: Vol. 2, a research annual* (pp. 71-109). Greenwich, CT: JAI Press.

Des Jarlais, D. C., Chamberland, M. E., Yancovitz, S. R. et al. (1984). Heterosexual partners: A large risk group for AIDS. *Lancet, 2*, 1346-7.

Des Jarlais, D. [as quoted in *New York Times*]. (1988, June 15). Spread of AIDS virus slows among drug users. (Write to author at New York State Division of Substance Abuse Services.)

Drucker, E. (1986). AIDS and addiction in New York City. *American Journal of Drug and Alcohol Abuse, 12*, 165-181.

Fineberg, H. V. (1988). Education to prevent AIDS: Prospects and obstacles. *Science, 239*, 592-596.

Fox, D. A., & Thomas, E. H. (1987/88, Winter). AIDS cost analysis and social policy. *Law, Medicine, and Health Care, 15*, 186-211.

Francis, D., & Chin, J. (1987). The prevention of Acquired Immunodeficiency Syndrome in the United States. *Journal of American Medical Association, 257*, 1357-1366.

Friedland, G. H., & Klein, R. S. (1987). Transmission of the Human Immunodeficiency Virus. *New England Journal of Medicine, 317*, 1125-1135.

Friedland, G. H., Saltzman, B. R., Rogers, M. F., Kahl, P. A., Lesser, M. L., Mayers, M. M., & Klein, R. S. (1986). Lack of transmission of HTLV-III/LAV infection to household contacts of patients with AIDS or AIDS-related complex and oral candidiasis. *New England Journal of Medicine, 314*, 344-349.

Gallo, R., Salahuddin, S., Popovic, M., Shearer, G., Kaplan, M., Haynes, B., Palker, T., Redfield, R., Oleske, J., Safai, B., White, G., Foster, P., & Markham, P. (1984). Frequent detection and isolation of cytopathic retroviruses (HTLV-III) from patients with AIDS and at risk for AIDS. *Science, 224*, 500-503.

Gerberding, J. L., Bryant-LeBlanc, C. E., & Nelson, K. (1987). Risk of transmitting the human immunodeficiency virus, cytomegalovirus, and hepatitis B virus to health care workers exposed to patients with AIDS and AIDS-related conditions. *Journal of Infectious Diseases, 156*, 1-8.

Guinan, M., & Hardy, A. (1987). Epidemiology of AIDS in women in the United States. *Journal of American Medical Association, 257*, 2039-2042.

Henderson, D., Saah, A., Zak, B., Kaslow, R., Lane, H., Folks, T., Blackwelder, W., Schmitt, J., LeCamera, D., Masur, H., & Fauci, A. (1986). Risk of nosocomial infection with human T-cell lymphotropic virus type III/lymphadenopathy associated virus in a large cohort of intensively exposed health care workers. *Annals of Internal Medicine, 104*, 644-647.

Hessol, N.A., Rutherford, G.W., O'Malley, P.M. et al. (1987). The natural history of Human Immunodeficiency Virus infection in a cohort of homosexual and bisexual men: A 7-year prospective study. *Abstracts, III International Conference on AIDS, Washington, DC, June 1-5, 1987*. Bethesda, MD: National Institutes of Health.

Institute of Medicine, National Academy of Sciences. (1986). *Confronting AIDS: Directions for public health, health care, and research*. Washington, DC: National Academy Press.

Institute of Medicine, National Academy of Sciences. (1988). *Confronting AIDS: Update 1988*. Washington, DC: National Academy Press.

Jaffe, H. W., Darrow, W. W., Echenberg, D. F., O'Malley, P. M., Getchell, J. P., Kalyanaraman, V. S., Byers, R. H., Drennan, D. P., Braff, E. H., Curran, J. W., & Francis, D. P. (1985). The Acquired Immunodeficiency Syndrome in a cohort of homosexual men: A six-year follow-up study. *Annals of Internal Medicine, 103*, 210-214.

Kingsley, L. A., Kaslow, R., Rinaldo, Jr., C. R., Detre, L., Odaka, N., VanRaden, M., Detels, R., Polk, B. F., Chmiel, J., Kelsey, S. F., Ostrow, D., &

Visscher, B. (1987). Risk factors for seroconversion to Human Immunodeficiency Virus among male homosexuals. *Lancet, 1,* 345-351.

Klug, R. (1986). Children with AIDS. *American Journal of Nursing, 86,* 1126-1132.

Koop, C. E. (1987a). Excerpt from keynote address. In B. Silverman & H. Waddell (Eds.), *Report of the Surgeon General's Workshop on Children with HIV Infection and Their Families* (pp. 3-5). Washington, DC: Public Health Service.

Koop, C. E. (1987b, June 18). [Testimony at hearing]. *AIDS and teenagers: Emerging issues. A Report of the Select Committee on Children, Youth, and Families, U.S. House of Representatives.* Washington, DC: U.S. Government Printing Office.

Koop, C. E. (1988). *Understanding AIDS.* (Available from Public Health Service, CDC, P.O. Box 6003, Rockville, MD 20850.)

Landesman, S. H., Ginzburg, H. M., & Weiss, S. H. (1985). The AIDS epidemic. *New England Journal of Medicine, 312,* 521-525.

Lui, K., Darrow, W. W., & Rutherford, G. W. (1988). A model-based estimate of the mean incubation period for AIDS in homosexual men. *Science, 240,* 1333-1335.

Mann, J. M. (1988, March). . . . for a global challenge. *World Health,* pp. 4-8.

Marzuk, P. M., Tierney, H., Tardiff, K., Gross, E. M., Morgan, E. B., Hsu, M., & Mann, J. J. (1988). Increased risk of suicide in persons with AIDS. *Journal of the American Medical Association, 259,* 1333-1337.

McKusick, L., Wiley, J., & Coates, T. (1985). Reported changes in the sexual behavior of men at risk for AIDS, San Francisco, 1982-84: The AIDS behavioral research project. *Public Health Report, 100,* 622-628.

Melbye, M. (1986). The natural history of Human T Lymphotropic Virus-III infection: The cause of AIDS. *British Medical Journal, 292,* 5-12.

Miike, L. (1987). *AIDS antibody testing: Testimony before the House Committee on Small Business.* Washington, DC: Office of Technology Assessment.

Moss, A. R., Osmond, D., Bacchetti, P., Chermann, J., Barre-Sinoussi, F., & Carlson, J. (1987). Risk factors for AIDS and HIV seropositivity in homosexual men. *American Journal of Epidemiology, 125,* 1035-1047.

National Institute on Drug Abuse. (1986). *Overview of the 1985 national household survey on drug abuse.* Rockville, MD: Public Health Service.

National Institute on Drug Abuse. (1987). *Trends in drug abuse related hospital emergency room episodes and medical examiner cases for selected drugs—DAWN 1976-1985* (DHHS Publication No. ADM 87-1524). Series H, No. 3. Rockville, MD: Public Health Service.

Office of Technology Assessment—Staff Paper. (1988, May). *How effective is AIDS education?* (DHHS Publication No. ADM88-6435). Washington, DC: U.S. Government Printing Office.

Petricciani, J. C., & Epstein, J. S. (1988). The effects of the AIDS epidemic on the safety of the nation's blood supply. *Public Health Reports, 103,* 236-241.

Piot, P., Plummer, F. A., Mhalu, F. S., Lamboray, J. L., Chin, J., & Mann, J. M. (1988). AIDS: An international perspective. *Science, 239,* 573-579.

Price, R. W., Brew, B., Sidtis, J., Rosenblum, M., Scheck, A. A., & Cleary, P. (1988). The brain in AIDS: Central nervous system HIV-1 infection and AIDS dementia complex. *Science, 239,* 586-591.

Public Health Reports. (1986). PHS plan for prevention and control of AIDS and the AIDS virus. Coolfont Conference. *Public Health Report, 101,* 341-348.

Pyun, K. H., Ochs, H. D., Duffort, M. T., & Wedgwood, R. J. (1987). Perinatal infection with Human Immunodeficiency Virus. *New England Journal of Medicine, 317,* 611-614.

Quinn, T. (1987). The global epidemiology of the Acquired Immunodeficiency Syndrome. In B. Silverman & A. Waddell (Eds.), *Report of the Surgeon General's Workshop on Children with HIV Infection and Their Families* (pp. 7-10). Washington, DC: Public Health Service.

Rogers, M. (1987). Transmission of Human Immunodeficiency Virus infection in the United States. In B. Silverman & A. Waddell (Eds.), *Report of the Surgeon General's Workshop on Children with HIV Infection and Their Families* (pp. 17-19). Washington, DC: Public Health Service.

Schuster, C. R. (1988). Intravenous drug use and AIDS prevention. *Public Health Reports, 103,* 261-266.

Schwartz, J. S., Dans, P. E., & Kinosian, B. P. (1988). Human Immunodeficiency Virus test evaluation, performance, and use. *Journal of the American Medical Association, 259,* 2574-2579.

U.S. House of Representatives. (1988a). *A Generation in Jeopardy: Children and AIDS. A Report of the Select Committee on Children, Youth and Families.* Washington, DC: U.S. Government Printing Office.

U.S. House of Representatives. (1988b). *AIDS and teenagers: Emerging issues. A Report of the Select Committee on Children, Youth and Families.* Washington, DC: U.S. Government Printing Office.

Watkins, J. D. et al. (1988). *Report of the Presidential Commission on the Human Immunodeficiency Virus Epidemic.* (Write: Presidential Commission, 655 15th Street NW, Suite 901, Washington, DC 20005).

Weiss, S. H., Goedert, J. J., Gartner, S., Popovic, M., Waters, D., Markham, P., Veronese, F., Gail, M. H., Barkley, W. E., Gibbons, J., Gill, F. A., Leuther, M., Shaw, G. M., Gallo, R. C., & Blattner, W. A. (1988). Risk of Human Immunodeficiency Virus (HIV-1) infection among laboratory workers. *Science, 239,* 68-71.

Wofsy, C. B. (1987). Intravenous drug abuse and women's medical issues. In B. Silverman & A. Waddell (Eds.), *Report of the Surgeon General's Workshop on Children with HIV Infection and Their Families* (pp. 32-34). Washington, DC: Public Health Service.

Wolensky, S. [as quoted in *Minneapolis Tribune*]. (1988, June 15). Test shows AIDS virus can be hidden longer than three years. (Write to author at: Northwestern University Medical School.)

Chapter 2

Strategies for AIDS Education and Prevention

Jeri Hepworth, PhD
Michael Shernoff, ACSW

"There have been as many plagues as wars in history—yet always plagues and wars take people equally by surprise" (Camus, as cited by Joseph, 1987, p. 15). Stephen Joseph, Commissioner of the New York City Department of Health, commented: "In the case of AIDS, the time for surprise is over. Rather than continuing to argue and skirmish over such peripheral issues as mandatory testing, the national debate must center upon a national prevention strategy that will work."

The significance of education and its role in AIDS prevention no longer can be debated. With no vaccine or cure for the human immunodeficiency virus (HIV) in the foreseeable future, education designed to affect behavior and attitudes is the most viable strategy to prevent the continued spread of HIV infection. To be effective, education must motivate people to recognize personal risk and to

Jeri Hepworth is Assistant Professor and Director, Behavioral Science, Department of Family Medicine, University of Connecticut, Asylum Hill Practice Center, 123 Sigourney Street, Hartford, CT 06105. Michael Shernoff is Adjunct Faculty, Department of Education, Gay Men's Health Crisis and Co-Chair, AIDS Task Force, American Orthopsychiatric Association. Correspondence to him may be addressed to: Chelsea Psychotherapy Associates, Suite 1305, 80 Eighth Avenue, New York, NY 10011.

The following persons contributed to the preparation of this chapter: Ann Welbourne-Moglia, Sandra Caron, Robert Walsh, Kenneth Davis, Ronald Moglia, Mary Bourne, Timothy Sankary, and Nelwyn Moore.

take action to change behaviors that put them at risk. It is difficult to achieve these goals because education about AIDS is not simply education about facts. Complex moral, ethical, and political controversies soon get triggered in even the most pragmatic of discussions about AIDS, resulting all too often in confusion, antagonism, and despair. Thus, educational efforts must take into consideration the intense feelings surrounding the topic of AIDS while seeking to motivate people to change their personal behaviors.

This educational task is not impossible. There is evidence that, with appropriate education and motivation, people engaging in high-risk behavior can and will modify these behaviors. For example, Winkelstein et al. (1987) have documented reductions of 60% or more in the prevalence of high-risk sexual practices associated with transmission of HIV for sexually-active gay men in San Francisco. The challenge for educators is to implement programs that will effect similar behavior and attitude changes in all groups. This chapter proposes principles to be followed in developing AIDS education, methods for building support for and implementation of AIDS educational programs, and specific educational and preventive strategies for various affected groups.

PRINCIPLES OF AIDS EDUCATION AND PREVENTION

The following principles should underlie the development of any AIDS education program:

1. *AIDS education is a public health issue affecting everyone and, hence, preventive education should be implemented immediately for everyone.* The entire population, including children, families, professionals, and the socially disenfranchised, have a right to AIDS education.

2. *AIDS education should be adapted so that it is culturally and developmentally appropriate for any given target audience.*

3. *AIDS education should be designed and implemented by professionals who are trained in* sexuality education, substance abuse education, small-group and community process, racial and ethnic variations, and individual and family dynamics.

4. *AIDS education should include factual information about the*

disease and provide a forum for discussion that will help people incorporate these facts into their lives. Therefore, AIDS educational programs must include opportunities for individuals to ask questions and to explore their attitudes and emotional reactions. Discussion of alternatives empowers participants to take personal preventive measures to avoid AIDS infection.

5. *AIDS education should emphasize risk behaviors which cause the spread of HIV.* It is important to concentrate on high-risk behaviors rather than on membership in high-risk groups. Labeling populations at high-risk is an effective epidemiological tool but is not an appropriate educational goal because it leads to blaming and to denial of personal risk among persons not defining themselves as members of such groups. Although targeting specific risk groups can be helpful in educational planning, the emphasis of any presentation must be on the full range of at-risk behaviors which allow transmission of HIV.

6. *AIDS educational programs in public schools must be taught as part of a comprehensive health program.* All school children have a right to be informed about AIDS transmission and prevention. Comprehensive health programs must be developed ensuring that children at every grade level are introduced to developmentally appropriate information concerning sexuality, substance abuse, and AIDS. Two AIDS education curricula designed for use in the public schools have received particularly positive reviews from educators (see Brick, 1987): *Teaching AIDS: A Resource Guide on AIDS* by Quackenbush and Sargent (1986) and *AIDS: What Young Adults Should Know* by William Yarber (1987b). Also see *SIECUS Report*, July-August, 1987, for review of books, curricula, and media for AIDS and safer-sex education, and *Morbidity and Mortality Weekly Report*, Jan. 29, 1988, Volume 37, No. S-2, for "Guidelines for Effective School Health Education to Prevent the Spread of AIDS."

7. *All AIDS educational programs should include a component addressing the relationships among behaviors, values, and social responsibility.*

8. *All AIDS educational programs should include an evaluation component.*

BUILDING SUPPORT FOR AIDS EDUCATION

Educators proposing AIDS education are likely to encounter numerous questions and concerns from the community. These frequently arise during initial discussions about AIDS education programs and occur whether the programs are designed for children, adults, or special populations. Sample concerns and suggested responses are identified here, but must be tailored by the educator to meet the specific needs of his/her community:

Concern: "We don't have anyone with AIDS in our community" or "It isn't a problem in our community."
Response: Few communities are so isolated that they have no interaction with the larger society. Although direct experience with AIDS may come more slowly to some areas, it is a national problem. Pretending that it is not *our* problem will not be an adequate health defense against AIDS. Eventually, most people are going to know someone in their family or among their friends who is infected with HIV or has AIDS.

Concern: "Our community is too conservative for such a program on AIDS."
Response: Conservatism will not defend a community from AIDS. AIDS affects people without regard to political affiliation or moral stance. Education about transmission and prevention is needed by all persons in every community, and we must seek to develop a program that is consistent with the values of our community.

Concern: "How can you tell us something about AIDS when no one seems to know much about it?" or "How can you tell us anything about AIDS when the information is changing everyday?"
Response: It is true that the information base is expanding continually, but specific information about AIDS is known. Information about routes of transmission and modes of prevention is based on extensive study of persons with AIDS. By June, 1988, over 60,000 cases of AIDS had been reviewed. Evidence suggests that the routes of transmission remain consistent with previous knowledge. We are now able to identify risk behaviors and, hence, begin to reduce the spread of HIV infection. Rather than waiting in fear for all the an-

swers, it is to our advantage to use existing knowledge to halt the further spread of HIV.

Concern: "I'm afraid that if you come into my class and talk about AIDS, you'll give my students a negative view of sexuality."
Response: We teach people how to drive safely, including specific information on the dangers and risks of hazardous driving. So far, this has not resulted in a decreased number of drivers on the road. Teaching people how to take precautions to protect themselves and to make responsible choices is not providing a negative view. There are genuine risks and young people have a right to know how to deal with them.

Concern: "If we institute AIDS education programs in this community, people will think we have a problem with AIDS."
Response: All communities have or will have a problem with AIDS. We educate about immunizations against whooping cough, polio, and other infectious diseases. Education and support for research on these diseases has made them a minor threat to community health.

Concern: "Don't you think this kind of information will hurt or psychologically damage our children?"
Response: Much of the information about AIDS is alarming. However, there is no way to shelter children, even very young ones, from the media or conversations at home, school, and among friends. Even when a topic is not discussed, children learn about the emotional significance of the topic by the way adults dismiss or respond to it. The best way to protect children is to provide them with facts in a calm and thoughtful way.

Concern: "We already know all there is to know about AIDS from the media."
Response: Television, radio, newspapers, and other publications have been an important source of information about AIDS. However, for many people, either too little or too much information is provided. The media tends to polarize issues and to stress sensational aspects, sometimes leaving people with more fear than knowledge. The media seldom provides an opportunity for one to ask questions, and yet we need a chance to discuss our concerns and

questions with others. Educational programs provide this interactive possibility.

Concern: "How can I have you talk about AIDS, when I've never talked to my class about sex?"

Response: AIDS is a public health problem. Discussion of AIDS can begin in this context and then move on to include sexuality education. Basic sexual education is essential if students are to become familiar with their bodies and how to care for them. There is probably a Family Life Education program in your community on which to build. If not, now is the time to establish such a program.

Concern: "I don't need to know about AIDS because I'm not in a 'high-risk' group. I'm not 'promiscuous', a homosexual, an IV drug user, a hemophiliac, or a blood transfusion recipient."

Response: If one is planning to live a life totally without sexual activity, to never have a blood transfusion, and to never know anyone who is HIV positive, one may not need to know anything about AIDS. However, the projected number of persons who will become infected with HIV indicates that millions of families in thousands of communities will be affected directly by AIDS. Many more people will be concerned and affected indirectly as communities evolve humane ways to care for persons with AIDS and HIV infection. Finally, since public policy decisions about health practices, treatment, and health-care financing will need to be made, AIDS will continue to affect all persons in this country for some time to come.

Concern: "I think it is important for young people to know about AIDS, but how can we teach them appropriate values?"

Response: It is impossible to educate about any subject without transmitting values. It is important that parents, educators, and communities determine what values will be taught and how these values can be transmitted best. In education about AIDS, the educator also is teaching the person to assume responsibility for his/her own safety. Because the educator cannot know the exact moment at which a person will need this information, it is best to give persons enough knowledge to make informed decisions as needed.

Concern: "The problem really isn't that bad" or "The media has blown this all out of proportion."

Response: AIDS is a major public health problem in the United States and worldwide. Although AIDS was first recognized in this country in 1981, by June, 1988, over 60,000 people had developed AIDS and over 35,000 had died (CDC, 1988). By 1991, it is projected that 270,000 persons will have developed AIDS in the United States. Until a cure for AIDS is discovered, or a vaccine against the AIDS virus is developed, the numbers of those infected will continue to rise. The situation is so alarming that in May, 1988, Surgeon General C. Everett Koop made an all-out effort to educate everyone in the United States about the dangers of AIDS. In a pamphlet sent to every home in the country, Koop (1988) advocated that middle-school students—those entering their teens—learn how to protect themselves against the AIDS virus and that basic health education start as early as possible.

Concern: "If young people get information about AIDS and 'safer sex,' you're going to put ideas in their heads, and they'll go out and try these things."

Response: We do not believe that AIDS education promotes an unhealthy interest in sexual topics. There are no data indicating that increased knowledge is correlated with increased sexual behavior. Developmentally-appropriate education about AIDS enables people to make more humane and knowledgeable decisions for themselves. These decisions may save their lives.

Family professionals can serve by encouraging AIDS education, helping to consolidate educational efforts by bringing together persons already involved in such efforts, and facilitating presentation and discussion of information. A particularly important role will be to raise community consciousness regarding the fact that AIDS impacts whole family units, not just isolated individuals, and that families include biological members as well as significant others involved with the infected individual.

Despite general agreement about the tragic consequences of AIDS, there is much disagreement and concern about prevention and education. If not handled carefully, these concerns may lead to dysfunctional controversy, further postponement, and even prevention of educational efforts. The following guidelines may be helpful in building community support for AIDS education:

1. *Document that there is wide public support for AIDS education and prevention programs*: A recent national survey indicates that Americans view AIDS as the nation's most serious health problem (News Service Reports, June 16, 1988). Surgeon General Koop, Secretary of Education Bennett, and President Reagan all went on record in support of efforts to educate and prevent AIDS. Further, a 1987 Gallup poll indicated that over 67% of adults favored sex education in the public schools (grades 4-8), including discussion of AIDS.

Building support for AIDS education programs begins by helping community members realize that they are not alone in wanting such programs. The controversy, if it occurs, can then center around the more important questions: (a) What will be taught? (b) Who will teach it? (c) How will it be taught? and (d) To whom will it be taught?

2. *Know the facts about AIDS*: There is a great deal of myth, misinformation, and public panic about AIDS. One consequence of this is more myth, misinformation, and immobilizing behavior and, in turn, less education and prevention. To counter this, each educator must know the significant facts about AIDS. These include current local, state, national, and international epidemiology (e.g., number of cases, number of deaths, racial and gender breakdowns) and the modes of transmission and prevention. Present and future projections for the particular community are very useful in gaining support and reducing denial.

3. *Utilize community models to organize programs*: Community organizational skills include utilizing existing resources, identifying pertinent people for support, assessing needs, and finding the additional resources necessary to initiate and carry out the educational efforts. This work includes identifying and consulting with the respected leaders in the community and meeting with them individually and in groups to identify concerns, areas of expertise, and local resources. It is important that these meetings recognize the existing work of AIDS educators in the community so that there is no implied competition or disparagement of efforts already in progress.

Family professionals, for example, may identify a more narrow educational focus (e.g., parent education) that will complement existing public health educational efforts.

After identifying community needs and concerns, the organizational work may include identification of those who are sufficiently concerned about AIDS to work further, perhaps on a local task force. The task force may encourage and develop educational programs, serve as a clearing house for expertise, and act as a resource for the community and media. As programs are developed and implemented, continued input from other community groups will be necessary to maintain community support. The task force should not develop unique programs without consulting existing programs and knowledgeable consultants.

Each community will have different needs and concerns. AIDS education programs must be developed and implemented in ways which reflect and are sensitive to the unique characteristics of each community. If the community appears resistant to AIDS education, it is easy to become discouraged. However, awareness of majority and minority attitudes, cultures, and concerns is of central importance for educative success. The following will help ensure success: (a) *begin where the community is comfortable beginning*; (b) *go slowly and include many community leaders*; and (c) *listen to the concerns of the community and address these concerns thoughtfully and thoroughly*.

AIDS education can elicit strong feelings about sexuality, lifestyles, values, and death. It is extremely important for those in leadership roles to understand the power of these feelings, while working to develop educational programs which can be helpful. Listening and working at an appropriate pace is essential. AIDS is a frightening epidemic. Yet AIDS also gives us an opportunity to work together as members of a community — at local, state, national, and international levels — and to respond responsibly and with compassion.

STRATEGIES FOR PREVENTION OF HIV TRANSMISSION

Epidemiological data have demonstrated that HIV is transmitted by (a) having anal, vaginal, or oral sex with someone who is infected; (b) sharing IV drug needles and syringes with an infected person; and (c) transfer from infected mother to infant before or during birth (Koop, 1988). Since the initiation of antibody testing in Spring, 1985, the risk of becoming infected from a blood transfusion in the United States has been reduced to about 1 in 39,000 transfusions, thus removing this from a high-risk transmission category (News Service Reports, June 16, 1988).

The fact that AIDS is sexually transmitted will not stop most people from having sex with others. The fact that sharing needles shares AIDS will not prevent drug users from using drugs. Moral or not, legal or not, less drastic changes in behavior are easier to accomplish and, therefore, more effective prevention techniques. This section briefly identifies techniques which can prevent or significantly decrease the transmission of HIV and discusses how these can be taught to different groups of people, depending upon the kinds of high-risk behaviors in which they engage.

AIDS is a *behavior-bound* disease, spread primarily by high-risk behaviors and not by membership in any particular risk group. Therefore, effective AIDS prevention education must emphasize those specific *behaviors* that pose high risks for transmitting HIV rather than focus on particular groups of "at-risk" people (Palacios-Jimenez & Shernoff, 1988). This approach helps to identify public health issues without stigmatizing people for group membership. The overriding moral issue of the AIDS epidemic is saving lives, not restricting drug use or sexual conduct. Education about behavior communicates the message that anyone can get AIDS and that each sexually-active person can prevent the spread of HIV.

To best address the diverse subgroups within our population and maximize behavior change, the message of prevention and change must be given repeatedly, over time, and be relevant to the targeted audience. Thus, a variety of strategies and interventions must be developed to address the differing concerns and lifestyles of heterosexual men and women, gay and bisexual men and women, and people who use drugs intravenously (Palacios-Jimenez & Shernoff, 1988). Moreover, to maximize compliance, AIDS prevention messages should seek to achieve the smallest amount of behavioral change necessary to prevent HIV transmission. The following are behavioral strategies designed to prevent the sexual transmission of HIV.

Abstinence

Complete absence of any sexual contact with another person offers 100% protection from sexual transmission of HIV and, therefore, is a viable prevention option. However, this is not a practical option for most persons. The high rates of adolescent pregnancy and the alarming rise of sexually-transmitted diseases among adolescents demonstrate that simply telling anyone, particularly adolescents, to abstain from sex is not effective.

Educational strategies must recognize that adolescents are very likely to engage in some form of premarital sexual activity despite religious and parental disapproval. Developmentally, adolescence is a period when the individual is interested in exploring sexuality and the developing body. It is currently estimated that 28% of persons aged 12 to 17 are sexually active and that about 70% of teenage girls and 80% of teenage boys have had at least one coital experience (Yarber, 1987a). The challenge for parents and professionals is to help adolescents place their sexual exploration in a moral framework, find alternatives to sexual intercourse, set limits, care for their own bodies, and respect partners who are not ready for intercourse, while acknowledging the adolescent's desire to engage in some form of sexual activity. Given the prevalence of AIDS, this challenge must be addressed immediately.

Adults also may choose sexual abstinence as a prevention strategy, but this is not without problems. Some formerly sexually-active adults report feeling trapped into choosing celibacy as their only viable response to fears about contracting AIDS. Some remain sexually abstinent for a period of time and, as a result of this "enforced" celibacy, report feeling very anxious, angry, and/or depressed. Some are not able to remain celibate on an ongoing basis and so periodically resume sexual activity in ways that are highly risky. This kind of "diet/binge" behavior is mentally and physically dangerous to the individual and to sexual partners (Palacios-Jimenez & Shernoff, 1988).

The diet/binge pattern also has been documented in a study conducted with 140 gay and bisexual men in conjunction with the San Francisco Department of Public Health (Beeson, Zones, & Nye, 1986). A small percentage of participants reported that attempts to remain celibate as a way of avoiding exposure to HIV actually re-

sulted in unsafe sex when they no longer felt able to remain abstinent. These data raise concerns about celibacy as an effective AIDS
prevention strategy. It appears that for adults who have been sexually active, sustained abstinence usually is not a feasible alternative
and strategies are needed to permit them to be sexual in ways that
will not put them at risk for transmitting HIV.

Sexual Exclusivity

Some professionals counsel that monogamy with "an absolutely
trustworthy partner" is one way of preventing the spread of HIV.
This is absolutely true if both partners have not been exposed to
HIV. A problem emerges when monogamy is cited, along with
masturbation and celibacy, as the *only* options for preventing transmission of HIV (Crenshaw, 1987).

Kinsey's research in the 1940s (Kinsey, Pomeroy, & Martin,
1948) and Hunt's research in the 1970s (Hunt, 1974) demonstrate
that the concept of lifelong monogamy is a myth for over 50% of
heterosexual married couples in the United States. Thus, the problem with monogamy as an AIDS prevention strategy is evident.
Few people of any sexual orientation can be absolutely certain about
the drug use or sexual history of their sexual partners or of the past
partners of these partners. Moreover, HIV can have an incubation
period of several years or more. Therefore, high-risk sex with *someone*, in effect, is also sex with *everyone* with whom that person has
had sex in recent years. The problems with assuming monogamy are
increased when small groups of people who are presumed not to be
infected with HIV agree only to have sex with one another. The strategy of "safe-sex clubs" is further complicated by the uncertainty of
HIV testing, which is discussed later in this chapter.

Another risk of employing monogamy as an AIDS prevention
strategy is that some cultural biases allow husbands, for example, to
use prostitutes and still be "faithful." Another variation is heterosexually married but homosexually active men who do not view
their sexual activities with other men as making them "unfaithful"
(or homosexual). These behaviors pose significant risks to both
members of the couple. A sexually monogamous relationship, in
which both partners have never been exposed to HIV, remains a
reasonable prevention strategy for many people. However, because

over half of the married population admits to extramarital sexual relationships and one outside sexual experience could introduce HIV into a relationship, to rely on another's monogamy as protection against HIV infection carries some element of risk.

Reducing the Number of Sexual Partners

Many have suggested that reducing the number of sexual partners is one means of lowering the risk of HIV exposure (see Boffey, 1988). Because it does not account for the form of sexual behavior or the risk level of the partners, this is misleading. For example, it is less risky to engage in mutual masturbation with large numbers of individuals than to be the receptive partner in unprotected anal or vaginal intercourse with one person who is HIV antibody positive. Far more important than *numbers* of partners is the choice of behaviors with those partners and the choice of partners.

Three recent studies found no correlation between multiple sexual partners and seropositive conversion for women who were sexual partners of men seropositive for HIV (Cohen, Hauer, Poole, & Wofsy, 1987; Fischl et al., 1987; Padian et al., 1987). The majority of women who became infected did so after engaging in ongoing high-risk sexual behaviors with one partner who was seropositive. Thus, women who believe that having fewer sexual partners reduces their risk of contracting AIDS may be falsely reassured about their risk status if those few partners happen to have shared IV drug paraphernalia, to have had sex with other men, or to be HIV seropositive. Certainly, fewer sexual partners will reduce transmission of HIV, but only if those partners are HIV negative or there is use of "safer-sex" practices.

Safer Sex

"Safer sex" describes a broad range of sexual activities that do not allow transmission of HIV because there is no exchange of body fluids. The activities include flirting, fantasy, hugging, body rubbing, dry kissing, massage, showering together, mutual masturbation with "on me *not* in me" orgasms, and correct use of an intact condom or other barrier device. The latter includes anal or vaginal intercourse using a condom and a *water-based* lubricant, fellatio with a condom or restricting oral contact to only the penile shaft, and cunnilingus with a barrier rubber dam.

Couples can augment safer-sexual stimuli with specific erotic fantasies and body pleasuring designed to increase sensuality and sexual satisfaction. These methods include sexually explicit talk between partners and the use of vibrators or other sexual equipment. It is important that the same piece of equipment not be used by both partners and that precautions be taken to ensure that body fluids never come into contact with the partner's mucous membranes.

Safer sex as an AIDS prevention strategy has found widespread acceptance among gay men around the country. Evidence of this is the marked decline in rectal gonorrhea and hepatitis B rates reported all over the U.S., but documented in San Francisco (McKusick, Horstman, & Coates, 1985) and in New York City (Centers for Disease Control, 1984). Gay men who have learned to eroticize safer sex have discovered that changing patterns of sexual behavior need not result in boring or deprived sex lives.

The above success has prompted suggestions that safer-sex become the preferred or recommended prevention strategy for most people. Critics, however, note that persons who do not feel personally at risk of infection for AIDS may not be motivated to use safer sex techniques. It may be that gay men are willing to adopt safer-sexual practices precisely because most of them either know someone who currently has AIDS, or who has died from AIDS, and/or are worried that they could contract the virus. This has resulted perhaps in a segment of the population which is highly motivated to change its sexual behavior.

Some sexuality educators also express concern that safer-sex education will not affect behavior, claiming that "sexual arousal is much like alcohol intoxication—the first thing to go is judgment" (Crenshaw, 1987). Thus, people may neglect when aroused to use condoms, or to use them correctly, or to engage in other safer-sexual practices. Ingestion of alcohol and recreational drugs may reduce further one's ability to remain within risk-reduction guidelines. Therefore, AIDS prevention education should include education about the effects of drugs and alcohol on behavior and urge persons to reduce substance use prior to sexual activities.

In order to convince all sexually-active adolescents and adults to practice safer sex, the message needs to be broadly communicated that *anyone can get AIDS and AIDS is 100% preventable*.

Condoms

Condoms have been shown in the laboratory to block the passage of HIV (Connant, Hardy, Sernatinger, Spicer, & Levy, 1986), especially if they contain Nonoxynol-9, a spermicide shown to inactivate HIV (Hicks et al., 1985; Voeller, 1986). Only latex condoms should be used to insure protection against transmitting HIV. Condoms must be of high quality and must *not* be used with petroleum-based lubricants (e.g., Vaseline) that can cause latex disintegration (Voeller & Potts, 1985).

Some have touted condoms as a "magic bullet" for preventing AIDS. This is simplistic and not accurate. Because condoms may break or be used improperly, they have been shown to significantly *reduce* but *not eliminate* the transmission of HIV. Condom use is a form of *safer* sex but *not* absolutely safe sex.

Proper use of the condom must be taught and adhered to strictly. Because pre-ejaculate fluid may contain HIV, latex condoms must be put on before sexual intercourse. Condoms must be applied carefully, leaving a portion loose at the tip of the penis to collect the ejaculate if the condom does not have a receptacle tip. The condom should be unrolled all the way to the base of the penis. Once applied, all excess air should be squeezed out of the condom. If the condom is not lubricated with Nonoxynol-9, a small amount of this spermicide should be put inside the tip of the condom to provide a protective barrier in case of breakage. The shaft of the penis should never be lubricated before a condom is applied. To protect against the possibility of breakage, water-based lubricant containing Nonoxynol-9 also should be used on the outside of the condom for added protection.

Condoms should only be used once. To protect against spillage of fluids, they must be removed carefully. Excessive heat (e.g., storage in the dashboard of a car) or carrying condoms for many months in a wallet deteriorates the latex. Attention should be paid to the expiration date on the condom package. Using safer-sex guidelines (i.e., no exchange of body fluids), condoms should not be lubricated with saliva. Until there are more conclusive data, the most prudent assumption is that fellatio and cunnilingus pose risks for transmitting HIV and, thus, should not be performed without a barrier.

Because condoms work only when people use them consistently as well as properly, education must address people's attitudes about using condoms. Many men view condoms solely as birth control for adolescents or low-income persons. If a woman suggests that a man use a condom, he may respond angrily, thinking that she is rejecting him or that she is "loose."

The most common reason given for not using condoms is the argument that they interfere with sexual satisfaction and reduce sensitivity. Other complaints are that condoms are unnatural, messy, kill spontaneity, and are uncomfortable. These complaints can be addressed by helping people learn to eroticize condoms and to incorporate them into foreplay. A recent study of 27 heterosexual couples conducted at the University of Georgia demonstrated that teaching people to incorporate condoms sensuously into foreplay significantly enhanced attitudes toward condom use (Tanner & Pollack, 1987). Directly confronting negative attitudes toward condom use by education may result in increased usage (Darrow, 1974).

Men who are inexperienced about condom use can be encouraged to purchase a variety of different brands and types (e.g., unlubricated, lubricated with powder, wet-lubricated, ribbed, receptacle-tipped, plain-end) and to experiment using them when alone. Practice in putting on a variety of condoms and masturbating will increase comfort with condom use and help the individual learn which varieties are preferred. To learn how much stress condoms can take and how it feels when one is torn, practice should include breaking the condom while masturbating. These same activities can be used by couples who wish to learn how to use condoms together.

HIV Antibody Testing

The HIV antibody test is not a test for AIDS, but a test for antibodies to HIV. Antibody testing indicates whether a person has been exposed to HIV and whether one is at risk for transmitting the virus to others. The HIV antibody test does not determine whether the person will develop symptoms of ARC or AIDS or when such symptoms might appear. Learning one's antibody status and the status of prospective partners is thought, by some, to be a technique for preventing transmission of HIV. The problem with this method is that a person may have been inoculated with the virus but not seroconverted at the time of testing.

It has been assumed that the usual period between HIV infection and seroconversion is about 6 to 24 weeks. Recently, however, researchers in Finland identified men who did not test positive for HIV antibodies until 14 months after exposure (Kolata, 1987), and current research indicates that the virus can go undetected for several years ("AIDS can be," June 15, 1988). Thus, a person may be tested during the period between exposure and seroconversion, receive a negative test result, and be reassured falsely that he/she cannot transmit HIV to others. This lag time for seroconversion is a problem for programs, such as the More-Health Institute in San Francisco, which suggest that one way to prevent HIV transmission is to have sex only with persons holding certificates documenting negative antibody status.

Antibody testing has almost no role as an AIDS prevention strategy in high prevalence populations (i.e., gay men living in San Francisco or New York). In these areas, persons must assume that they or their sexual partners are already HIV infected and, therefore, practice safer sex. An exception to this would be the couple that has been sexually monogamous for 10 years, plans to remain sexually monogamous, and agrees to "confess" if either has another sexual partner. Another exception would be the couple that has been sexual partners for less than 10 years, has always practiced safer sex, but now wishes to be tested to discover if they can abandon safer sex with each other. Heterosexual couples who have not engaged in high-risk activities are unlikely to use safer sex very long when they believe that the likelihood of infection for either is low. Persons in such couples may wish to confirm their antibody status before removing restrictions on the kind of sex they can enjoy with one another.

There are many controversies surrounding antibody testing. A positive test result often results in feelings of guilt, anxiety, and depression. Some persons experience reactions severe enough to require psychotropic medication or psychiatric hospitalization

(Shernoff, 1987). Persons considering an antibody test are urged to obtain detailed information about the test from a sophisticated counselor, to consider their probable reactions to the test result, and to receive counseling about the implications, whether the result is negative or positive. Because there is much public concern about how test results may be used by health insurers, employers, and acquaintances, the antibody test always should be done anonymously or confidentially.

STRATEGIES FOR AIDS PREVENTION EDUCATION FOR SPECIFIC POPULATIONS

Providing adequate education about how to reduce the risks of contracting or transmitting HIV poses many challenges for professionals. One challenge is how to reach the many relevant and diverse segments of the general population, such as adult heterosexual singles, gay or bisexual men, men who have sex with men and do not identify with the gay community, adolescents, low-income women, and IV drug users.

Effective AIDS prevention education results in behavior change. In order to achieve behavior change, the following are necessary:

1. *People must recognize that AIDS can be a direct threat to them.* Often this occurs when someone with whom they identify gets ARC or AIDS or confides that they are seropositive for HIV. For heterosexual men, the group least likely to feel at personal risk, videotapes of heterosexual men who became infected from a female sexual partner are helpful.

2. *People must learn that AIDS is preventable and that they can act to protect themselves and their sexual partners from infection.* This requires a specific understanding of transmission and prevention techniques, explained in easily understood language. The idea can be conveyed that changing only a few specific behaviors results in reducing greatly the risks of transmission. Behavior change does not occur usually without attitude change and, to maintain behavioral changes, persons often need to address their feelings of anger, guilt, and loss.

3. *Everyone needs to believe that they can be content with the various lifestyle changes necessary to stop HIV transmission.* The

goal is for each person to believe that he or she can have a satisfying, risk-free sex life. Some people find the use of peer support an effective way to motivate and maintain change over time.

Peer support takes many forms. It occurs within a couple when the partners communicate appreciation that the other cares enough about both of them to avoid high-risk behaviors. It is present in mass media campaigns when celebrities or athletic stars promote condom use and discuss taking responsibility for one's personal health and partner safety. It often involves support groups in which people discuss fears and learn new methods from one another. An example of peer support is the gay community where safer sex has become the norm (Centers for Disease Control, 1985) and where a man who puts himself or partner at risk often finds himself without a sexual partner or ostracized by others.

Three levels of AIDS prevention education should be occurring simultaneously in the United States (Palacios-Jimenez & Shernoff, 1988). *Primary prevention* attempts to prevent the occurrence of any more new cases of HIV infection. Every person in this country should become informed about the exact transmission of HIV and the necessary acts for personal prevention. The use of AIDS education in schools to prevent transmission among newly sexually-active adolescents is a mode of primary prevention. Another positive example is the mailing of AIDS information by the U.S. Public Health Service to 100 million households in May, 1988 (Koop, 1988). A national campaign in England used billboards and the media to urge the British public "not to die from ignorance."

Secondary prevention is addressed to those who already have tested positive for HIV but are asymptomatic for any signs of active HIV infection, ARC, or AIDS. The goal is to prevent them from transmitting the virus to others and from re-exposing themselves to HIV or other infections that will weaken further their immune systems. Such persons need specific information on protection for themselves and their sexual partners. They often benefit from psychosocial support which explores the personal meanings and implications of seropositivity.

Tertiary prevention is for persons diagnosed as having ARC or AIDS and focuses on reducing, as much as possible, the disabling aspects of AIDS. Efforts should be made to help the individual participate as actively as possible in normal occupational, leisure, and social activities and to take an active role in his/her treatment by attending support groups and by learning about nutrition as well as techniques of stress management and relaxation. The goal is to maximize quality of life and to reduce fear, isolation, and helplessness (Macklin, 1988).

All educational presentations, whatever the level, should be guided by basic educational principles. Presentations should be tailored to the audience, recognizing the different types of information required by each. Information sessions should include time for questions and answers and be followed by small-group discussion. Some means should be provided for participants to ask embarrassing questions (e.g., provide paper and pencils and ask *all* participants to hand in at least one question). Anonymity is especially important when a question might reveal illegal or stigmatized behavior. The following sections discuss issues to be considered when developing educational programs for specific populations.

IV Drug Users

IV drug users are the second largest category of persons with AIDS, comprising more than one quarter of all documented cases of AIDS (CDC, 1988). IV drug users are the major source for heterosexual transmission of AIDS and, through pregnancy, the major route for transmission to infants. One study showed that 80% of male IV drug users have sexual relations with women who are not IV drug users (Institute of Medicine, National Academy of Sciences, 1986). Thus, drug users are at high risk for transmitting AIDS through sexual activity as well as through drug usage (Ginsburg, 1984). Prevention, therefore, must address both safer sexual activities and the drug-use behaviors which allow blood to be shared.

The illegality of drug use, and the lack of advocacy and community resources for drug users, make it especially difficult to develop educational and support groups for this population. The popular image of the IV drug user as an isolated, distrustful, self-destructive, criminal person with little concern for health makes some policy-makers loath to "waste" educative efforts on this group.

Contrary to the above stereotype, IV drug users are heterogeneous, representing all racial, ethnic, economic, and social-class groupings. There is a continuum from the occasional, nonaddicted users to those who must get a fix daily. Whereas a suburban user may be able to obtain a regular supply of clean needles, impoverished users may share needles because they have no equipment of their own, especially if they are youth just being initiated into IV drug use. This makes it doubly important to get information about the dangers of sharing "works" to adolescents prior to their potential exposure to IV drugs.

As has been repeatedly stated by the Public Health Service (e.g., Koop, 1987), even the smallest amount of infected blood left in a used needle or syringe can contain live AIDS virus which can be injected into the next user of those dirty implements. Most heroin users administer the drug intravenously and the majority of IV drug users share equipment (Levy et al., 1986). Needle-sharing is often part of the IV drug subculture, serving as a social bonding mechanism (Institute of Medicine, National Academy of Sciences, 1986).

Although there is diversity among IV drug users, there is at least one shared concern: IV drug use is illegal. Fear of police and the legal system are serious concerns and confidentiality is of utmost importance. Organizational techniques that might be effective within gay communities are likely to fail completely when used with IV drug users. Substance abuse counselors and IV drug users must be included in education programs to provide credibility for the programs, to develop peer contacts for drug users, and to assist with educational strategies and appropriate language.

In general, the benefits of not using drugs have not been adequate to pull users away from drugs. The question remains: Can the threat of AIDS be enough of a "push" to induce change? It is well known that behavior modification changes based on fear are not generally successful. Change is much more likely when the feared event immediately follows the behavior and when specific ways to avoid the feared event are clearly identified. Des Jarlais, Friedman, and Hopkins (1985) have expressed concern that the long latency period, the common flaunting of death by IV drug users, and the ambiguity of AIDS-related symptoms all impede the perception of AIDS as a highly personal threat. However, in the 3 years since the

Des Jarlais article was written, AIDS has received a great deal of media attention. It is hoped that the media coverage and the increased awareness of deaths from AIDS will have an impact on those using IV drugs. Indeed, even at the time of writing, Des Jarlais and his associates concluded from AIDS awareness data and from reduction of needle-sharing that IV drug users are capable of modifying their behavior and that risk reduction had begun to occur (Des Jarlais et al., 1985).

The educational message useful to drug users is that they can take charge of their own lives. This is best accomplished by supporting programs designed to assist in stopping the use of IV drugs. Hence, the expansion of drug treatment programs is essential. It may be necessary to convince legislators that the cost of expanding drug treatment programs is far less than the cost of treatment for one person with AIDS and many times less than the cost of treating those persons whom he/she might infect. It is noteworthy that the President's Commission on the HIV Epidemic has recommended establishment of a "treatment on demand" system for IV drug users, thus making treatment immediately available for any IV drug user who seeks it (Watkins et al., 1988).

If people are not able or willing to stop using IV drugs, at least they should be encouraged to stop sharing needles or be taught disinfecting procedures. After a "set" is cleaned of any residue, soaking for 30 minutes in one cup of water with two tablespoons of bleach will disinfect the set (Illinois Department of Public Health, 1986).

The AIDS prevention campaign in Amsterdam, The Netherlands, is based on the principle that if curing drug addiction is not possible, a situation should be created that greatly reduces the risk that the addict will become HIV infected or transmit the infection (Buning, Coutinho, van Brussel, van Santen, & van Zadlehoff, 1986). The Amsterdam program includes a publicity campaign in which leaflets are distributed, an exchange system for needles and syringes, and a system of distribution of condoms to prostitutes who are drug addicts.

A study of drug users by the Street Research Unit in New York City reported that the period after drugs have been obtained is characterized by an intense desire to use these drugs. If new needles are available during this period, they will be used, but, if not, whatever needles are handy will be used (Des Jarlais et al., 1985). Therefore, the availability of clean needles would seem to be a very effective AIDS prevention strategy. Implementation of this strategy, of course, requires the modification of laws regarding the sale or exchange of needles.

Ordinarily, education about drug use and AIDS should begin in schools and at home. However, IV drug use is concentrated primarily among people who no longer attend school. Hence, other places for information and presentations are needed, including churches, clinics, jails, "on the street," soup kitchens, "hangouts," and workplaces. Former or present drug users can be very helpful in identifying locations for information and referring people to information centers.

Community telephone hotlines are excellent information sources when confidentiality is important. Hotlines allow for more probing questions of the caller and encourage more open disclosure by the caller. People with poor reading skills and partners or friends of IV drug users who may be afraid to go to public meetings or special group sessions can get answers more readily over a hotline. A number of very successful community hotlines are in existence (e.g., a hotline in Rochester, New York, staffed by volunteers who have training in drug and sex education). When setting up an AIDS hotline, a call to an existing program can be very useful.

Traditionally, the medical community has referred drug users to substance abuse counselors. Although there is value in this specialized network, which often includes former substance users, there is still a need for the general medical community to become thoroughly educated about HIV and drug use. Some IV drug users, especially occasional users, may prefer to obtain information, counseling, and treatment from a neighborhood doctor than from a substance abuse clinic. Information about IV drugs and AIDS left in waiting rooms may be read by family members or sexual partners of the IV drug user. Hotline telephone numbers and other drug treatment resources should be available in all doctors' offices and hospital waiting areas.

Gay and Bisexual Men

A variety of strategies have helped gay and bisexual men successfully change their sexual behaviors (e.g., McKusick et al., 1985). In New York City, the Gay Men's Health Crisis, the oldest and largest AIDS service-provider organization in the world, has run a monthly all-day "Safer Sex Forum" for gay men for the last several years. More than 300 men have attended these forums at any given time. The workshop includes a medical overview of AIDS provided by a physician, information about transmission of HIV and condom use, a sexually-explicit safer-sex video, and a discussion about eroticizing safer sex. Small discussion groups throughout the day allow participants to talk about feelings, concerns, and questions.

A half-day workshop on "Eroticizing Safer Sex" has been presented nationally, drawing as many as 500 men at one time in large metropolitan cities and college campuses (Palacios-Jimenez & Shernoff, 1986). In these workshops, participants are encouraged to explore their feelings about changing sexual behaviors, allowing them to consider and role-play safer-sexual options and new skills. The Institute for the Advanced Study of Human Sexuality in San Francisco has conducted similar safer-sex workshops on the West coast, including a training program for Safer Sex Instructors.

Another kind of strategy are safer-sex "Tupperware-style" parties, given for small groups of men in private homes. Conducted by volunteers from local AIDS service organizations, the forums provide opportunities for people to obtain information and to raise their concerns. Participants are urged to host similar gatherings, with the organization providing materials and a facilitator.

The success of these campaigns in gay male communities provides a variety of models for conducting effective AIDS prevention programs for all people. A crucial task is to translate these models into effective programs for educating heterosexuals. Examples are workshops advertised for heterosexual persons or couples on "Sexual Enhancement and Sexual Enrichment in the Age of AIDS."

A very difficult population to reach is the closeted heterosexually-married, homosexually-active man. Because they do not generally identify themselves as gay, these men do not attend workshops advertised for gay men. They are the people most likely to engage in anonymous, homosexual sexual activity and the least likely to discuss their sexual activities with their heterosexual partner. Therefore, new interventions must be developed and advertisements distributed in places where men are meeting for anonymous sex, including movie houses, bookstores, and rest stops.

Women

Approximately 8% of the people with AIDS in the U.S. are women (CDC, 1988). About half of these are intravenous drug users. Of the increasing numbers who are infected via sexual contact, the majority are partners of intravenous drug users. A minority are partners of bisexual men, hemophiliacs, and blood transfusion recipients. Almost three-quarters of women with AIDS are poor, minority, and from the inner city (Joseph, 1987). The particular goals of AIDS education for women include helping them protect themselves when their partners are HIV-infected and helping them prevent HIV transmission to their unborn children.

The Hyacinth Foundation, New Jersey's state-wide AIDS service provider organization, reports that the sexual partners of low-income women often refuse to wear condoms. Some women who have attempted to insist on condom use have been raped, battered, or threatened with the loss of their relationship. One woman told a Hyacinth staff member, "I either have a roof over my head and a meal ticket by having sex with him without a condom or I'm out on the street!" (M. Nichols, personal communication, November 6, 1987).

In response to this situation and to insure the highest degree of protection from HIV, the Hyacinth staff suggest that women use multiple forms of barrier contraception that also employ Nonoxynol-9. Using a diaphragm or cervical cap in addition to foam or a sponge soaked in the spermicide and having a man use a condom would provide the highest level of safety. But when the man refuses to wear a condom, using at least one, and preferably two, means of barrier contraception that includes Nonoxynol-9 provides some degree of protection for the woman.

Women who are at risk of pregnancy or who are pregnant need to be informed that HIV infection can be transmitted to infants in utero or at birth and possibly through breast milk. Moreover, women who are HIV-infected need to know that pregnancy increases their risk of developing AIDS. This means that education and counseling efforts must be mounted at family planning clinics and in medical offices as well as via the public media. The decision of whether to risk pregnancy or to continue a pregnancy will be a difficult one for many HIV-infected women and, especially, for women who are partners of HIV-infected men but not yet infected themselves.

Lesbians are not at high risk of contracting or transmitting HIV unless they have used IV drugs, received blood transfusions or blood products between 1979 and 1985, or have had unsafe sexual contact with persons in risk groups. If they are planning pregnancy through donor insemination, they may wish to request that their donor be tested for HIV antibody. Because of the lag between infection and antibody development, the test should be done twice prior to insemination with a period of 3 to 6 months between tests and with the donor practicing safer sex during this period. If a woman has reason to believe that she may be HIV-infected, or is engaging in activities that place her at risk, she should not allow her menstrual blood or vaginal secretions to enter her partner's body through the mouth, rectum, vagina, or broken skin.

Prostitutes

Prostitution places the prostitute and partners at increased risk of exposure to all sexually-transmitted diseases, including AIDS. Many prostitutes feel that the risk must be accepted in order to survive financially. The safest strategy, of course, is to find another line of work. If, however, a prostitute intends to continue work, the most efficient strategy at this time is the strict use of condoms with spermicides and other safer-sex practices wherever practical. In Nevada, where prostitution is legal, all prostitutes are regularly tested (although this does not protect against the time lapse between infection and the development of antibodies). A similar law was proposed in Los Angeles, requiring all masseuses to have regular antibody tests in order to be licensed. This was defended on the grounds that, although prostitution is illegal, it cannot be eliminated and safety may be increased through regulation. These approaches address the risk posed to the customer by infected prostitutes, but fail to offer any protection to the prostitutes themselves. Because some prostitutes also obtain HIV from IV drug use, strategies aimed at preventing the spread of HIV via shared needles are necessary for this group.

Many persons have called for mandatory antibody testing of convicted prostitutes. Testing would enable prostitutes and public health officials to have knowledge of their antibody status and enable states to impose criminal penalties for continuing prostitution when infected with HIV. Although threatening, it is unlikely that these measures alone would be effective in eliminating the spread of HIV via prostitution. Continued education for all people about the risk of unprotected sexual intercourse with multiple partners is essential.

Prisoners

Recent public policy decisions by the Reagan administration and the American Medical Association have advocated mandatory AIDS testing for all prison inmates. This reflects the high rate of drug use, the limited availability of "works" for injections, some consensual homosexual behavior, and the potential for criminal assault or rape in the prison setting. The legal and ethical responsibility of prison officials to protect the health and safety of inmates includes protecting against possible transmission of HIV by infected prisoners and protecting HIV-infected prisoners from persecution and possible violence by guards and other inmates. Whether the disposition of isolation or restricted activities will be justly handled is dependent on the personal qualifications, knowledge, and prejudices of the warden and the particular penal system.

Education of prison personnel must address issues related to provision of appropriate counseling and ways to ensure safety of prison inmates and staff from infection and discrimination. Educational programs for inmates must consider the diversity of racial and ethnic persons in the penal system and adapt to the cultural beliefs and languages of the represented populations.

Transfusion Recipients and Hemophiliacs

All transfusion recipients and hemophiliacs who received blood or blood products between 1979 and May, 1985 need to receive counseling about whether they wish to be tested for HIV. Unless results of the antibody test are negative, it is prudent to assume possible exposure to HIV and to take the same precautions as those recommended for persons with HIV (see below).

Persons with HIV Infection

Persons with HIV infection should avoid all activities which might allow them to be exposed further to HIV and all activities which could transmit HIV to others. Persons with HIV, therefore, should not donate blood, semen, or body organs. In addition, they should not share IV drug needles or participate in unsafe sexual activities. Because there is much uncertainty about how or why persons with HIV develop AIDS, it is very important that persons with HIV avoid any behaviors which might further weaken their immune systems or increase their risk of infectious diseases. (For further discussion, see chapter on Therapeutic Issues in this volume.)

Families and Partners of Persons with HIV

Families, lovers, partners, and members of households of persons with HIV infection require education about contact with the infected person and prevention of infection for themselves (see NIMH, 1986). Education must present clearly the evidence that casual contact, including sharing of food, eating utensils, bathrooms, telephones, and other common household contact, does not allow the spread of HIV (see the chapter on the HIV Epidemic in this volume). Education also should include information about the illness, possible progression of the disease, and risks and treatment strategies for the person with HIV infection. Partners of all persons with AIDS should avoid the exchange of body secretions by conscientious use of the prevention techniques described in earlier sections. However, touching, kissing, and hugging do not pose dangers of transmission to uninfected persons. The health risks, in fact, are greatest for the person with HIV infection who may need to be protected from other infectious illnesses.

Because responses to the diagnosis of AIDS or report of seropositivity are affected by cultural and individual fears and beliefs, facts alone are not sufficient. Educational efforts for families and friends must include ample opportunity for people to raise repeated questions, to learn that their fears or beliefs are normal and common, and to discuss the numerous, often ambivalent, feelings that naturally occur (see chapter on Therapeutic Issues for further discussion). Educative strategies must address these concerns in appropriate forums. Strategies identified earlier, including the use of anonymous written questions, small-group discussion, viewing of videos and films, and presentations given by family members of persons with AIDS are all useful techniques.

Family and partners will provide the majority of care to persons with AIDS throughout the course of illness. Families need to be educated about the normal course of the disease and its concomitant psychosocial effects, issues related to their roles as caregivers and support persons, and the possible long-range benefits that can occur when family members and friends pull together in such a crisis. As with anyone caring for persons with AIDS, families will benefit from outside support themselves. Thus, education for families should focus on identification of family stressors and possible resources and support services.

The profound impact of AIDS on family units is beginning to be documented by clinical programs, such as the AIDS Project of the Ackerman Institute for Family Therapy (Walker, Mohr, Patten, Kaplan, & Gilbert, 1988), and to be described in the popular and professional press (e.g., see Frierson, Lippman, & Johnson, 1987; Peabody, 1986; Tiblier, 1987; Walker, 1987). Because of the tendency for families to feel isolated in their crisis, such information can be particularly helpful for those involved in the home care of persons with AIDS. Efforts should be made to educate the community to the need for support groups and services for families, friends, and partners. The Visiting Nurses and Hospice of San Francisco is developing the AIDS Family Network, a computer listing of families of persons with AIDS willing to be contacted by other families for support and assistance (see chapter on Resources in this volume). Information about local support groups can be obtained from local AIDS information services, the National AIDS Hotline sponsored by the Centers for Disease Control and the American Social Health Association (800-342-7514), and the National AIDS Network (202-347-0390).

Racial and Ethnic Minorities

AIDS is an "equal opportunity disease." Since the first reports of AIDS, Blacks and Latinos have been overrepresented in proportion to their numbers within our society. As of mid-1988, Blacks represented 11.7% of our population but 26% of AIDS cases; Latinos represented 6.4% of the population but 15% of the AIDS cases (CDC, 1988).

Even when one controls for regional differences, minorities are disproportionately represented in every risk group with the exception of hemophiliacs and transfusion recipients (CDC, 1988). About 75% of the approximately 5,000 women and 1,000 children who had been diagnosed with AIDS nationally as of June, 1988, were Black or Latino. In 1988, AIDS was the leading cause of death of Black and Latino women aged 25-29 in New York City. Of the 2,694 heterosexually-transmitted AIDS cases (excluding gay and bisexual men, IV drug users, and transfusion recipients) reported as of June, 1988, over 80% were Blacks and Latinos, five times larger than that of the White population (499 cases).

Reporting of Asian/Pacific Islanders and Native Americans is incomplete and believed to be masked by misdiagnosis or inaccurate reporting of the disease by community health providers. It is suspected that the less sophisticated medical treatment centers are not accurately diagnosing AIDS and, hence, the proportional percentages for minority groups may be even higher than the above figures indicate.

Racial minorities historically have underutilized health care for a variety of reasons. Factors such as low socioeconomic status, high unemployment, and limited access to education and health-care resources suggest that AIDS will continue to affect minority people disproportionately. Minority persons frequently are uninsured for health services, do not seek medical treatment until an illness is critical, and have to travel many miles to receive such care. Clinical evidence indicates a survival rate for Blacks with AIDS of 8 months compared to 18 to 24 months for Whites (NIMH, 1986). This survival rate discrepancy is at least partially attributable to inadequate health-care services offered too late to an already vulnerable population.

Future projections of the impact of AIDS on minority people are alarming, especially considering the present rates and the time lag between infection and onset of the disease. Until 1987, there were no educational efforts supported by the federal government addressing educational needs for minorities, particularly those in cities.

Because of differences in cultural values and practices, preventive and educational models used in White communities cannot be transferred automatically to the many diverse minority populations. For example, the image of AIDS as a disease for gay, White men has been a significant obstacle to education and support within minority communities. It will be important to draw upon knowledge about health practices and educational efforts that have been effective for different ethnic groups in the past. Culturally sensitive educational models using language and practices appropriate to each segment of the minority community are required. Too often, literature used by gay organizations has been modified minimally, or not at all, and inappropriately distributed to "straight" minority populations. These groups were so baffled by the terminology and found the material so embarrassing that they frequently avoided any discussion of its content or existence.

Schools, churches, social organizations, recreation facilities, and health and welfare agencies need to develop strategies of intervention for reaching various ethnic and minority groups. The more that members of the respective ethnic communities are involved in program development and actual presentation of content, the less resistance there will be to the educational message. Health fairs, clinics, educational groups, political block clubs, and indigenous community leaders trained as AIDS Education Resource People should be utilized. For example, to insure availability of support systems and sensitivity to ethnic lifestyles and language, testing sites for antibody status should be staffed by members of the local community. Because maintaining confidentiality will become more difficult when neighbors are also care providers, confidentiality must be a special priority for these community-based testing sites.

Lastly, ministerial associations, actors, sports figures, musicians, artists, and business people from the particular ethnic group being targeted can be used to promote AIDS information and risk-reduction procedures via newspapers, magazines, television, radio, and other media resources. Where possible, persons with AIDS and their family members should be involved in all planning and presentations. Not only does this permit the sharing of expertise, but it encourages the audience to identify more quickly and more compassionately with the epidemic and its issues.

GENERAL GUIDELINES FOR PARENTS

Education about AIDS is tied inextricably to education about sexuality. A child's sex education begins at birth and continues with the many silent lessons about sexuality transmitted daily by parents. These include how the infant is held, stroked, and soothed as well as the quality of care received. All impart major messages affecting the child's emerging sexual attitudes and behaviors (Calderone, 1966). The most crucial aspects of sexuality education are taught unconsciously as children observe parents model loving or non-loving behavior and foster positive or negative self-esteem (McCary, 1978). It is not only specific sexual knowledge, but also general attitudes about self and relationships that determine a child's later sexual behavior. Therefore, sexuality education is viewed optimally as an integral part of the total parent-child relationship.

Although both professionals and parents agree that parents have the primary responsibility for sexuality education in their children's lives, most parents feel unprepared. The following factors, delineated by Clark and Wilson (1983, pp. 3-4), are believed to inhibit open communication about sexuality between parents and their children:

1. Parents may perceive themselves as uninformed about sexuality and, therefore, unable to give their children adequate information.
2. Parents are often uncomfortable discussing sexual topics.

3. Parents often lack the necessary communication skills to discuss sexuality. They may not have learned about sex from their parents and, therefore, do not have models for teaching.
4. Parents often are unable to separate their desire to control and/or discipline their children's sexual behavior from their desire to give information.
5. Children, especially adolescents, may feel anxious when parents initiate a discussion on the subject of sexuality and, hence, not respond when the subject is raised.
6. Children and parents may have difficulty acknowledging each other as sexual beings.
7. Parents who are aware of changing sexual mores may be unsure about what they believe and what values they want to communicate to their children.

As the child's most influential sexuality educators, parents have specific needs for educational support systems. Educators, clinicians, clergy, and medical personnel increasingly are recognizing the need to provide training in sexuality education to parents. The challenge of such programs is to bridge the gap between what parents need to do and what they are able to do. Strategies necessarily will be as diverse as the groups they serve. Goals also may vary but should, at least, include helping parents to:

1. *Clarify attitudes* — Instead of learning specific answers to specific questions, parents need to clarify for themselves their and society's attitudes concerning (a) self as a sexual being, (b) the goals of sexuality education, and (c) the significance of their role as sexuality educators. It is important that parents become as comfortable as possible with the content so that they can present sexual and AIDS-related information to their children in as calm and neutral a manner as possible. Without such preparation, parents will transmit inadvertently their anxiety to their children.

2. *Increase knowledge* — Parents need information about (a) child growth and development and the essential needs governing behavior at each stage in the child's life, (b) the uniqueness of their individual child, and (c) methods of teaching. Finally, in order to help their child focus on prevention, parents must be knowledgeable

concerning basic and recent facts about human sexuality, sexually transmitted diseases, and AIDS.

3. *Improve communication skills* — Parents must become more skilled about communicating attitudes and knowledge to their children. Basic communication skills include giving and receiving feedback, active listening, sending consistent messages, and interpreting body language. To apply these skills, parents need (a) guidelines for specific ages, (b) resources, such as age-appropriate literature, and (c) supervised practice in such communication.

Whatever their views about sex education, parents have the opportunity and responsibility to protect their children from the fatal disease of AIDS. Although many parents feel unprepared to talk with their children about AIDS and sexuality, parents must overcome their discomfort in talking about sexual health. The following suggestions from *How to Talk to Your Children About AIDS* (Moglia & Moglia, 1986) may make the job easier:

1. The most important step that parents can take is to begin the conversation themselves. Children do not always ask questions about sex or AIDS, and so adults often must initiate the discussion.

2. It is likely that a child already has heard the word "AIDS." A good time to open the discussion might be following a television program or after reading a newspaper or magazine article that discusses AIDS.

3. Do not put off talking to children about sexual health. As children grow, they want to know more and more about their bodies, relationships, and sexuality, but they often become more self-conscious about discussing these topics. Begin discussion before the child goes to school and continue it into adulthood. It is never too late to begin.

4. Throughout discussions, try not to confuse the horrible consequences of getting AIDS with the positive joys of human sexuality.

5. When talking with a child about sexuality and AIDS, parents are also telling children that they care about their health and happiness. This can be one of the greatest joys of parenting.

The parent-child interaction should provide for the child's social, emotional, and cognitive needs in a developmentally appropriate way. Because every child is unique, the pattern and rate at which a child will pass through the normal developmental stages will vary. *Therefore, education should be designed so that it is generally age-appropriate, but tailored to the individual needs of one's own child.* The following information may be helpful in establishing guidelines.

Age-Appropriate Strategies for Preschool Children (0-4)

Preschoolers are interested in basic body functions and learn about their world through play activities. Educational activities should include correct use of anatomical words for body parts and accurate but simple answers to all inquiries. Very young children do not understand abstract concepts. Preschoolers demonstrate an early childhood form of logic, often resulting in unique interpretations of complex topics. Therefore, any specific reference to AIDS should reassure a child that this is something that s/he does not have to worry about at this time. The best thing a parent can do at this age is to set a tone in which children learn to feel free to ask any questions about their bodies, health, and sexuality. This lays the groundwork for open, honest discussion that can continue at the older ages.

Age-Appropriate Strategies for Early School-Age Children (5-9)

Early school-age children can learn fairly complicated concepts about life when the explanation utilizes concrete examples from their own life. Thus, if a child cuts him/herself, this may be a time to explain how "dirt and other things that can make you sick may get into your blood if we are not careful." The home and school can assist each other in helping the child to grasp the concepts of infection and illness, and parents and teachers can inform one another if a child seems particularly interested in or disturbed by information about AIDS. Because, at this age, children are aware of individual differences, all learning experiences should be multi-cultural and nonsexist.

Age-Appropriate Strategies for Pre-Teens (9-12)

Pre-teens begin to anticipate the physical, emotional, and social changes of puberty. They are primarily concerned about their bodies, their appearance, and what is "normal." For some young people, this also marks the beginning of dating and possibly the start of early sexual experiences and experimentation with drugs.

Peer pressure to experience sex and drugs can begin early, making it important that parents talk with their children about sexuality and AIDS even if they believe their children are not involved in these activities. Concerned parents must insure that their children have relevant information *NOW*. Because of the changes associated with puberty, pre-teens are very curious about sexual behaviors and need to be given accurate information about terms such as intercourse, homosexuality, oral and anal sex, and condoms. This may seem like a difficult task, but it is far better for children to have accurate information than to pretend knowledge to friends or to make decisions based on incomplete information. Discussions between parents and pre-teens enable parents to learn from their children and, in turn, to teach their children desired values.

Age-Appropriate Strategies for Adolescents (13-19)

Significant developmental concerns for adolescents include establishing identity and self-esteem through relationships with peers. Part of the process involves separating from parents and becoming more independent. Social pressures to try sexual experiences or to experiment with drugs are very strong. Therefore, at this age, regardless of the kind of sexual or drug experiences of the adolescent, *all* young people must be told the following: (a) *All* sexual relations that are not with a long-term and trusted partner should make use of "safer sex" practices. This includes no exchange of semen and vaginal secretions, the use of condoms and Nonoxynol-9 for all types of intercourse, and the use of condoms with fellatio. The responsibility for safer sex lies with both partners. (b) Avoid sexual contacts of any kind with persons known or suspected to be HIV-positive, IV drug users, or involved sexually with multiple persons. (c) Avoid having sex with multiple partners. (d) Do not use drugs and do not share hypodermic needles or razors.

At all developmental levels, children need the support and counsel of parents. Discussions about drugs, sexuality, and AIDS enable parents and children to learn that they can talk with one another about difficult moral and ethical concerns. The long-term benefits of these discussions extend beyond protecting children and adolescents from exposure to HIV.

SPECIAL ISSUES FOR PROFESSIONAL EDUCATION

Professionals, whether they are health-care providers or educators, have special needs for education about AIDS. Recent surveys of physicians have documented insufficient knowledge and negative attitudes about AIDS. Lewis, Freeman, and Corey (1987) reported that a majority of surveyed physicians in California had neither the knowledge nor did they practice the behaviors needed to care for patients concerned about or ill with AIDS. Kelly, St. Lawrence, Smith, Hood, and Cook (1987) stated that "As members of the general community, physicians are no doubt susceptible to many of the same stereotypes and biases as the community at large" (p. 789). Thus, education for professionals must begin by providing accurate information about epidemiology, transmission, and prevention of HIV infection.

As is the case for all audiences, providing facts alone is not a sufficient form of education. Like all people, the responses of health-care professionals inevitably reflect cultural and moral belief systems. Surveys by Kelly et al. (1987) and Lewis et al. (1987) document the prevalence of stereotyping and negative attitudes about persons with AIDS among health-care providers. They conclude that health-care professionals must examine their own attitudes about AIDS and persons who have AIDS, and seek to change those attitudes that permit stigmatization and prevent optimal care.

An educational program for health-care providers developed by Hepworth, Schmidt, and Sinapi (1986) includes three components: a factual presentation about epidemiology and transmission of HIV, a videotaped personal account from a person with AIDS, and a small-group discussion format in which the personal implications of the facts are considered. The latter is stimulated by a discussion questionnaire containing controversial statements about AIDS. An important goal is to help professionals recognize that personal values affect decisions regarding health care and policy. Any such educational program must include presenters who are aware of recent facts and available resources, willing to recognize their own limitations of knowledge and bias, and able to encourage self-questioning by group participants. A team of presenters is recommended.

CONCLUSION

The most effective AIDS educational programs present prevention options so that people may choose the most appropriate strategies for protecting themselves and others from transmission of HIV. Such strategies include stopping all behaviors which allow blood to blood contact, changing sexual behaviors to include condoms and other "safer sex" techniques, and consideration of abstinence, sexual exclusivity, and antibody testing.

AIDS requires that Americans in the late 1980s profoundly alter their sexual attitudes and behaviors. It is important to find a way of relating sexually which acknowledges our positive sexuality while expressing it in ways which foster health and relationship. The era of "no-fault sexual activity" is gone. To insure that the American public is protected against HIV, the content and means for education about sex for children and adults must change as well. Information about sexuality, substance use and abuse, and AIDS must be taught explicitly, beginning at an early age, and within a moral and ethical context which stresses decision making, personal values, and social responsibility. The explicit message should be "Do not have sex before you are ready to take responsibility for your sexual behavior and the effect it will have on your body, your health, and your life." Further tragedies from AIDS can be avoided by teaching all Americans how to protect themselves and their loved ones.

Robert Kennedy is said to have stated, "Few will have the greatness to bend history, but each of us can work to change a small portion of events. And in the total of those acts will be written the history of a generation." Hopefully, it will be written that our generation of educators, family professionals, and parents responded to the challenge of AIDS prevention with courage, compassion, integrity, and realism.

REFERENCES

"AIDS can be silent infection for years." (1988, June 15). *The Post-Standard* (Syracuse, NY), p. A-7.

Beeson, D., Zones, J., & Nye, J. (1986). *The social consequences of AIDS antibody testing: Coping with stigma*. Paper presented at the annual meeting of the Society For the Study of Social Problems, New York, NY.

Boffey, P. M. (1988, April 22). Researchers list odds of getting AIDS in heterosexual intercourse. *New York Times*, p. A-1, A-18.

Brick, P. (1987). Curricula reviews: AIDS education for survival. *SIECUS Report, 15*(6), 16-17.

Buning, E. C., Coutinho, R. A., van Brussel, G. H. A., van Santen, H. W., & van Zadlehoff, A. W. (1986). Preventing AIDS in drug addicts in Amsterdam. *Lancet, 3*, 435.

Calderone, M. S. (1966). Sex education for young people — and for their parents and teachers. In R. Brecher & E. Brecher (Eds.), *Analysis of human sexual response*. New York: New American Library.

Centers For Disease Control. (1984, June 11). Declining rates of rectal and pharyngal gonorrhea among males — New York City. *Morbidity and Mortality Weekly Report, 33*, 295-297.

Centers for Disease Control. (1985, October 11). Self-reported behavioral change among gay and bisexual men — San Francisco. *Morbidity and Mortality Weekly Report, 34*, 613-615.

Centers for Disease Control. (1988, June 27). *AIDS Weekly Surveillance Report*. Atlanta, GA: CDC.

Clark, T. S., & Wilson, P. M. (1983). *Sexuality education strategy and resource guide: Programs for parents*. Washington, DC: Center for Population Option.

Cohen, J., Hauer, L., Poole, L., & Wofsy, C. (1987). *Sexual and other practices and risk of HIV infection in a cohort of 450 sexually active women in San Francisco*. Paper presented at the Third International Conference on AIDS, Washington, DC.

Connant, M., Hardy, D., Sernatinger, J., Spicer, D., & Levy, J. (1986). Condoms prevent transmission of AIDS-associated retrovirus. *Journal of the American Medical Association, 255*, 1706.

Crenshaw, T. (1987, April). AIDS Update: Condoms are not enough. *Newsletter, American Association of Sex Educators, Counselors, and Therapists, 18*, 20-22.

Darrow, W. W. (1974). Attitudes toward condom use and the acceptance of venereal disease prophylactics. In *The condom: Utilization in the United States*. (Reprint #00-2634). Washington, DC: U.S. Government Printing Office.

Des Jarlais, D. C., Friedman, S. R., & Hopkins, W. (1985). Risk reduction for the Acquired Immunodeficiency Syndrome among intravenous drug users. *Annals of Internal Medicine, 103*(5), 755-759.

Des Jarlais, D. C., & Hopkins, W. (1985). "Free" needles for intravenous drug users at risk for AIDS: Current developments in New York City. *The New England Journal of Medicine, 23*, 1476.

Fischl, M., Dickinson, G., Scott, G., Klimas, N., Fletcher, M., & Parks, W. (1987). Evaluation of heterosexual partners, children, and household contacts of adults with AIDS. *Journal of the American Medical Association, 257*, 640-644.

Frierson, R. L., Lippman, S. B., & Johnson, J. (1987). AIDS: Psychological stresses on the family. *Psychosomatics, 28*, 65-68.

Gallup Poll Source Document. (1987, March 22).

Ginzburg, H. M. (1984, March/April). Intravenous drug users and the Acquired Immune Deficiency Syndrome. *Public Health Reports, 99*(2), 206-211.

Hepworth, J., Schmidt, P., & Sinapi, L. (1986, May). *Psychosocial aspects of AIDS: A component of family medicine education.* Workshop presented at the annual meeting of the Society of Teachers of Family Medicine, San Diego.

Hicks, D. R., Martin, L. S., Getchell, J. P., Heath, J. L., Francis, D. P., Mc-Dougal, J. S., Curran, J. W., & Voeller, B. (1985). Inactivation of LAV/HTLV-III infected cultures of normal human lymphocytes by Nonoxynol-9 in vitro. *Lancet, 2*, 1422.

Hunt, M. (1974). *Sexual behavior in the 1970s.* Chicago: Playboy Press.

Illinois Department of Public Health. (1986). *About AIDS and shooting drugs.* Springfield, IL: Author.

Institute of Medicine, National Academy of Sciences. (1986). *Confronting AIDS: Directions for public health, health care, and research.* Washington, DC: National Academy Press.

Joseph, S. C. (1987, August 15). Toward a national AIDS prevention strategy. *Hospital Practice, 22*(8), 15-16.

Kelly, J. A., St. Lawrence, J. S., Smith, S., Hood, H. V., & Cook, D. J. (1987). Stigmatization of AIDS patients by physicians. *American Journal of Public Health, 77*, 789-791.

Kinsey, A., Pomeroy, W., & Martin, C. (1948). *Sexual behavior in the human male.* Philadelphia: Saunders.

Kolata, G. (1987, October 3). Test for AIDS may fail to detect infection for more than a year. *New York Times*, p. 1.

Koop, C. E. (1987). *Surgeon General's Report on Acquired Immune Deficiency Syndrome.* Washington, DC: Public Health Service.

Koop, C. E. (1988). *Understanding AIDS.* HHS Publication No. (CDC)HHS-88-8404. Rockville, MD: Public Health Service.

Levy, N., Carlson, J. R., Hinrichs, S., Lerche, N., Schenker, M., & Gardner, M. B. (1986). The prevalence of HTLV-III LAV antibodies among intravenous drug users attending treatment programs in California: A preliminary report. *The New England Journal of Medicine, 314*(7), 446.

Lewis, C. E., Freeman, H. E., & Corey, C. R. (1987). AIDS-related competence of California's primary care physician. *American Journal of Public Health, 77*, 795-799.

Macklin, E. D. (1988). AIDS: Implications for families. *Family Relations*, *37*, 141-149.

McCary, J. L. (1978). *McCary's human sexuality*. New York: D. van Nostrand & Co.

McKusick, L., Horstman, W., & Coates, T. J. (1985). AIDS and sexual behavior reported by gay men in San Francisco. *American Journal of Public Health*, *75*, 493-496.

McKusick, L., Horstman W., Coates, T. J., Wiley, J., Stall, R., Saika, G., Morin, S., Charles, K., & Conant, M. A. (1985, November/December). Reported changes in the sexual behavior of men at risk for AIDS, San Francisco, 1982-1984: The AIDS research project. *Public Health Reports*, *100*, 622-629.

Moglia, R. M., & Moglia, A. W. (1986). *How to talk to your children about AIDS*. New York: New York University and Sex Information and Education Council of the United States.

National Institute of Mental Health. (1986). *Coping with AIDS: Psychological and social considerations in helping people with HTLV-III infection*. Rockville, MD: U.S. Dept. of Health and Human Services.

News Service Reports. (1988, June 16). *The Post-Standard* (Syracuse, NY), p. A-6.

Padian, N., Marquis, L., Francis, D., Anderson, R., Rutherford, G., O'Malley, P., & Winkelstein, W. (1987). Male-to-female transmission of HIV. *Journal of the American Medical Association*, *258*, 788-790.

Palacios-Jimenez, L., & Shernoff, M. (1986). *Facilitator's guide to eroticizing safer sex: A psychoeducational workshop approach to safer sex education*. New York: Gay Men's Health Crisis.

Palacios-Jimenez, L., & Shernoff, M. (1988). AIDS: Prevention is the only vaccine available. *Journal of Social Work & Human Sexuality*, *6* (in press).

Peabody, B. (1986). *The screaming room*. San Diego: Oak Tree Publication.

Quakenbush, M., & Sargent, P. (1986). *Teaching AIDS: A resource guide on AIDS*. Santa Cruz, CA: Network Productions.

Shernoff, M. (1987, October). Pre- and post-test counseling for individuals taking the HIV antibody test. *SIECUS Report*, *16*(7), 10-11.

Tanner, W., & Pollack, R. (1987, November). *The effect of condom use and sensuous instruction on attitudes toward condoms*. Paper presented at the annual meeting of the Society for the Scientific Study of Sex, Atlanta, GA.

Tiblier, K. (1987). *Intervening with families of young adults with AIDS*. In M. Leahey & L. Wright, *Families and life-threatening illness*. Springhouse, PA: Springhouse Corporation.

Voeller, B., & Potts, M. (1985). Has the condom any proven value in preventing the transmission of sexually transmitted disease — for example, Acquired Immune Deficiency Syndrome? *British Medical Journal*, *291*, 1196.

Voeller, B. (1986). Nonoxynol-9 and HTLV-III. *Lancet*, *3*, 1153.

Walker, G., Mohr, R., Patten, J., Kaplan, L. S., & Gilbert, J. (1988). AIDS and family therapy. *The Family Therapy Networker*, *12*(1), 22-43, 76-79, 81.

Walker, L. A. (1987, June 27). What comforts AIDS families. *The New York Times Magazine*, pp. 16-22, 63, 64, 67, 78.

Watkins, J. D. et al. (1988). Interim report of the Presidential Commission on the Human Immunodeficiency Virus Epidemic: Chairman's recommendations — Part I. *Journal of Acquired Immune Deficiency Syndromes*, *1*(1), 69-103.

Winkelstein, W., Samuel, M., Padian, N., Wiley, J., Lang, W., Anderson, R., & Levy, J. (1987). The San Francisco Men's Health Study: III, Reduction in human immune deficiency virus transmission among homosexual/bisexual men, 1982-1986. *American Journal of Public Health*, *76*, 685-689.

Yarber, W. L. (1987a). School AIDS education: Politics, issues, and responses. *SIECUS Report*, *15*(6), 1-5.

Yarber, W. L. (1987b). *AIDS: What young adults should know*. Reston, VA: American Alliance for Health, Physical Education, Recreation and Dance.

Chapter 3

Therapeutic Issues When Working with Families of Persons with AIDS

Kay B. Tiblier, PhD
Gillian Walker, ACSW
John S. Rolland, MD

The HIV epidemic has placed new demands on all of us. With insufficient education about AIDS, many families and communities have experienced panic. Persons with AIDS are sometimes separated from their families of origin or from traditional systems of support. The disease, itself, is a roller-coaster, often necessitating alternating hospital stays and home-care periods. Families with an HIV-infected member—sometimes two or more—experience multiple stressors. The psychological and relationship issues generated or stimulated by the disease are often as debilitating as the disease itself.

Kay B. Tiblier is Associate Clinical Professor, School of Nursing, University of California, and Lecturer in Sociology at San Francisco State University, San Francisco, CA. Her mailing address is 554 Liberty Street, San Francisco, CA 94114. Gillian Walker is Co-Director, AIDS Project, Ackerman Institute for Family Therapy, 149 East 78th Street, New York, NY 10021. John S. Rolland is Assistant Professor, Department of Psychiatry, School of Medicine, Yale University, New Haven, CT, and Medical Director, Center for Illness in Families, 400 Prospect Street, New Haven, CT 06511.

Special appreciation is extended to G. Mary Bourne, ACSW, President and Director of Training, Minnesota Institute of Family Dynamics, who made thoughtful contributions to this chapter.

Persons with AIDS and their families frequently need help (a) to adjust to the life-threatening diagnosis; (b) to deal with fears of contagion; (c) to accept the sexual orientations of family members; (d) to cope with stigma and discrimination; (e) to manage conflict among family members and significant others; (f) to confront a time-limited push for reconciliation; (g) to prepare for loss and bereavement; (h) to shift family roles; and (i) to provide necessary care and negotiate with external systems (Tiblier, 1987).

"Business as usual," focusing solely on the patient and utilizing only the traditional service model, will not meet the enormous pressures AIDS puts on the entire family and the health-care system. Professionals who work with persons with AIDS will be unable to provide adequate care without the help of the client's family, friends, and significant others. The quality of care and the extent to which available resources are utilized will depend largely on the values, attitudes, and wisdom of the relevant professionals.

By describing the emotional needs of HIV-infected persons and their families, this chapter seeks to promote increased compassion and cooperation among all available caring people — extended family, lovers, friends, volunteers, and professional caregivers — as a way of providing necessary support to the men, women, and children touched by AIDS. AIDS provides an opportunity to heal many distressed families and relationships (e.g., see Gilbert, 1988; Kaplan, 1988; Mohr, 1988; Patten, 1988; and Walker, 1988). This chapter provides insights essential to effective psychotherapeutic treatment of HIV-infected families and helpful to persons working in a range of caregiving and human service fields.

BASIC PRINCIPLES OF CARE

Three principles are basic to the development of human services for HIV-infected persons and their families. These should underlie the organization and provision of treatment and services, regardless of setting. They are as follows: (a) The family, both biological and functional, must be the basic unit of care in the psychotherapeutic treatment of persons who are HIV-infected; (b) care is best provided by a multi-disciplinary team; and (c) universal access to treatment must be available for all persons affected directly or indirectly by HIV infection.

Family, as used in this context, is defined in broad, comprehensive terms. It includes family of origin, family of procreation, cohabiting couples, friendship networks, and the "emergent family" of caregivers which often evolves following an AIDS diagnosis. In some instances, more than one member of the family is HIV-infected. All members of the family, whatever its configuration, will need educational information and support to deal with the emotional stressors accompanying AIDS. It is important to define the family broadly, so that all available resources are utilized and to assure that sufficient help is provided to the emotional system affected by the disease.

Care is best provided by a multi-disciplinary team working in close, nonhierarchical cooperation. Such a team could include physicians, nurses, discharge planners, nutritionists, respiratory and physical therapists, chiropractors, acupuncturists, psychologists, social workers, clergy, and family therapists working together with family, friends, and volunteers. Such an approach mitigates against burnout for professionals as well as family caregivers and provides the widest range of options when addressing the multitude of medical, psychological, social, spiritual, and economic issues associated with AIDS. The Ackerman Institute for Family Therapy, Gay Men's Health Crisis in New York City, Shanti in San Francisco, and Visiting Nurses and Hospice of San Francisco provide excellent models (see addresses at end of chapter). Hospice, for example, requires one person from the family or friendship network to serve as coordinator of emotional care, with others in the health-care team providing the care for which they are best equipped.

In an epidemic of this scale and intensity, convenient and universal access to treatment is essential. Care planning must occur on a local, state, and federal level, with attention to the international concerns raised by the World Health Organization. Universal access to care is not only humane, but a public health model with long-term cost effectiveness.

Individuals who work with persons with AIDS are not unanimous regarding the importance and appropriate role of the family of origin in treatment. Some maintain that often it is not possible to re-

connect the person with AIDS with the family of origin and to seek
to do so creates too much stress for someone who is already vulnerable. Others argue that the family of origin is of critical importance
and that it is essential to address alienation at almost any cost. The
material which follows attempts to sample both sides of this debate,
reflecting a desire to use resources wherever they can be found and
to avoid polarization along theoretical lines. Our hope is to show
the ways in which family can be valuable to the treatment team and
to the person with AIDS, and to identify the needs of families at
each of the points on the HIV-infection continuum from initial diagnosis to grieving and reorganization after death. Because of the
range of family forms which may present themselves, and the diversity of family cultures, the impact of the family's characteristics on
its reaction to AIDS and to treatment will be discussed first.

POSSIBLE CLIENT-FAMILY CONFIGURATIONS

The Male Couple

It is not unusual in some geographic areas for gay couples to have
one partner with full-blown AIDS and the other with asymptomatic
HIV infection. This may have the effect of putting a boundary
around the couple, increasing their dependence on each other. In
some couples, the healthier partner may feel imprisoned by the
needs of the ill partner, having fantasies of escape but feeling too
guilty to abandon his lover.

Illness may cause some couples to break normal relations with
their families of origin in order to avoid sharing their diagnoses,
thus leaving them devoid of that potential support. Others may
mend ties to parents or siblings and, in doing so, perhaps stress the
relationship between the lovers. As the illness progresses and additional caretakers and support groups appear on the scene, the person
with AIDS may become emotionally involved with them or find it
easier to confide in them than in his partner. This may either increase the distance between the couple or serve to diffuse tensions
so that they may be more easily resolved (e.g., see Carl, 1986;
Patten, 1988; Walker, 1987). In many cases, the original couple

dynamics will be disturbed by the diagnosis, as, for example, when the ill person was the more dominant in the relationship.

Whether or not one or both persons are infected, most gay couples will be at least indirectly affected. They may find themselves hesitant to terminate their relationship because of fear about reentering the potentially dangerous singles world. They may struggle with the question of whether to be tested for seropositivity. They are likely to have friends who are ill and to experience periods of grieving and concern.

Heterosexual and Bisexual Couples

As the disease spreads among the larger population, there are an increasing number of heterosexuals who are seropositive and who will eventually contract AIDS. The heterosexual couple with an infected member may feel isolated because the support systems typical of the gay community are not perceived as being so readily available to them. The couple may try to conceal the disease from the community in which they live. To their associates, AIDS may symbolize sexual infidelity or promiscuity, deviant drug use or homosexuality, and, hence, subject them to the same discrimination often experienced by gay couples.

When the disease is only manifest in one partner and where there is the risk of possible infection of the other, issues regarding HIV antibody testing may arise. There must be a careful exploration of the meaning of the test results for the individuals and the potential impact of these on the relationship. Issues of potential false positives, vulnerability to possible social disclosure, the stress of uncertainty, and the possibility of infecting others must be considered. Some individuals and couples are not comfortable with ambiguity, whereas others decide that they do not need information about their serostatus in order to make decisions about their relationship or their interaction patterns. Whatever the decision, it is important that the counselor present options rather than impose solutions and that the couple be educated regarding responsible sexual practices.

In some instances, a wife first learns of her husband's bisexuality when she learns of his AIDS diagnosis. Intense feelings of rage, shame, confusion, and betrayal may result. Simultaneously, she must come to terms with her husband's sexual orientation and its implications for her own health and the relationship. Since most persons are relatively uninformed about the nature of bisexuality, the wife's initial rage may be followed by acute depression and a sense of failure as a partner (see Coleman, 1982a and b; Weeks, 1985). The therapist needs to help the couple understand the complex underlying issues, give some positive meaning to their relationship as it has existed, and help them make decisions about the immediate future.

HIV-Infected Parents of Young Children

When a parent has AIDS, issues of shame and fear of social ostracism often force the family into patterns of secrecy which can threaten normal relationships. Children may hear parents discussing AIDS but be punished if they use the word, disclose their fears to outside persons, or ask too many questions. Family feuds may determine to whom the person with AIDS discloses the illness, and family members may find themselves alone with the knowledge that another family member is dying. In refusing to tell others, old family coalitions may be preserved and historical splits perpetuated (e.g., see Penn, 1983).

As children begin to sense that their parent is dying, they need the security of knowing who will care for them. When the parent can no longer provide care, children need help in adjusting to new caregivers and changed circumstances. Even if these issues are addressed before the parent dies, complex battles over custody may arise later. For example, a mother, infected by an addicted father, dies. Later, the father, who is still alive, and both sets of grandparents enter the fray and compete for custody of the children. Family therapists are well positioned either to calm down and reintegrate the complex network of alliances and coalitions or to encourage emotional cutoffs and sabotage the family's potential to provide support. In a crisis situation, it is important to observe the fine line between helping the family and further fragmenting it (see Walker, 1987).

Parents of Adult Children with AIDS

Parents of adult children with AIDS often need therapeutic help (for potential responses of parents to AIDS in their children, see Cleveland, Walters, Skeen, & Robinson, 1988; Tiblier, 1987). When an adult child is gay, issues resulting from the family's homophobia need to be resolved and any tendencies toward emotional cutoff reversed if the family members are to make peace with one another. In addition to the grief which any parent feels upon the loss of an adult child (see Shanfield, Benjamin, & Swain, 1984), many parents of gay persons report feelings of guilt and failure. There may be hesitation to turn to their friends and other family members for support. If they are the parents of the caregiving partner, their attitude toward the partner with AIDS may be a complex amalgam of compassion for their own child's loss and rage at his partner for placing their child at risk. In crisis it is easy to place blame on another person, thus forming a family-of-origin coalition against the outsider "third party" (see Coleman, 1982a and b; Myers, 1982; Patten, 1988).

As the AIDS epidemic progresses, stories are told of families for whom the experience of caring for an ill member has been one of transformation. Frequently, the family find that the love they feel for the dying family member transcends the individual prejudices they have held about that person's lifestyle. They come to see the individual as a person, not as a member of a socially deviant group, and, in so doing, develop better capacities to relate on an intimate level with one another.

For example, one suburban family with seven children described their experience of caring for a dying gay son as transforming each family member. The mother said that she stopped caring about what people thought and was determined to shed the trivia of her life about which, heretofore, she had cared too much. A sister became politically active on behalf of AIDS patients and their families. A rather detached physician son said that caring for his brother changed the way he worked with patients, bringing emotion, understanding, and sensitivity to his practice. A rebellious youngest son reported that being with his dying brother had drained the anger out of him and freed him to pull his life together. All of the family members were able to turn the caregiving experience into one of growth rather than alienation and went on to speak openly in the community about their experiences.

Extended Family Systems

The crisis of AIDS often sharpens family battles and increases conflicts. In one case, a married woman, who was extremely attached to her family of origin, felt forced to choose between caring for a dying brother and her marriage. When she considered caring for him at her mother's home, her husband complained. When she decided instead to bring him home, her husband left. When the brother died, the wife immediately turned her attention to taking care of another brother who was also at risk for AIDS, and the husband cut off entirely.

In order to better understand or anticipate the reaction of a family to an AIDS diagnosis, the therapist should note where the family is in its developmental lifecycle and explore how the family has organized itself in current and previous generations around illness and loss (e.g., see Carter & McGoldrick, 1988; Combrinck-Graham, 1985; Duvall, 1977; Herz, 1988; McGoldrick & Walsh, 1983; Moos, 1984; Neugarten, 1976; and Rolland, 1987b and c). A multi-generational illness-oriented genogram can help to elicit discussion of individual members' experiences in their families of origin with unexpected crises and to describe the family configuration prior to diagnosis, including relevant splits, alliances, collusions, and cutoffs (see McGoldrick & Gerson, 1985). This process also will help the therapist gain insight into how the person with AIDS is positioned in the family and how the family positions itself vis-à-vis that person. The skillful family therapist utilizes the family resources to increase its caregiving ability, to reduce conflicts which may stress the person with AIDS, and to bring the family to a measure of peace and resolution (e.g., see Boszormenyi-Nagy & Spark, 1973; Framo, 1976). An ideal outcome, perhaps seldom realized, is for a family to provide ongoing support for its dying member and to emerge stronger than it was before AIDS.

To identify and mobilize more easily the resources in the family system, the family therapist can construct a social network map in the first or second interview. By carefully charting the available persons who know and care about the patient, one can identify caregiving resources which can be utilized to provide home-care and alternatives to inpatient hospitalization (see Auerswald, 1968; Imber-Black, 1988). Collaterals who might provide service include distant kin, neighbors, clergy and rabbis, members of the family's congregation, as well as more closely related family members who may not have been considered by the patient or staff. To create and organize such family or family-like support structures, the family therapist must utilize the broadest possible definition of "family system." This system can then function both for the person with AIDS and for the family itself as it moves through illness and death and into the succeeding phase of reorganization.

SOCIOLOGICAL VARIABLES AFFECTING RESPONSE TO AIDS

Ethnicity, race, religion, and social class are important determinants of the way a family experiences any illness, including AIDS. These factors create the larger context into which the foregoing family configurations fit, much like a series of concentric circles. These variables help to determine the composition of the caregiving unit, the meaning attached to AIDS and those behaviors which may have led to infection, the ways a given family handles illness and death, and the bereavement and reorganization processes which necessarily must follow. Ethnic, racial, and religious groups differ in the definition of (a) what constitutes a family, (b) the responsibility of families in caring for ill members, (c) the family member chiefly responsible for care, and (d) the role of the extended family in times of crisis.

Ethnicity

AIDS may disrupt the way the family traditionally provides for caretaking at the time of illness (see McGoldrick, Pearce, & Giordano, 1980, for an excellent discussion of family ethnicity). Because of the shame associated with AIDS, the diagnosis may not be shared with the usual caregiving family members. The person with

AIDS, for instance, may designate a sibling who seems more tolerant of his/her lifestyle to replace the mother as caregiver, thus upsetting the normal family hierarchy. An example is a Latino family in which the mother was the caregiver and the matriarch. Two of her sons still lived at home and she was closely involved with her children, her daughter's husband, and her grandchildren. Although, normally, all crises would be routed to the mother for resolution, when one of her IV drug-using sons was diagnosed with AIDS, the siblings decided to shield her from the exact nature of his illness. Caregiving fell to the oldest daughter who left her husband and returned home to take care of her brother and to handle the relationship between him and his hospital caregivers. When, at last, his condition deteriorated to the point that the mother had to be told, she exhibited severe symptoms of heart failure and had to be hospitalized in the same hospital as her son. Her children apparently had surmised correctly that an AIDS diagnosis, with its accompanying shame, guilt, and finality, would devastate their mother. Her years of dealing with a son's drug addiction had in no way prepared her for the despair that this diagnosis would bring. It is characteristic of many family structures that the oldest daughter would take over the caregiving function of the mother in times of stress, and that her loyalty to family of origin would outweigh her loyalty to her own marriage.

In some ethnic groups, rigid definitions of who is the designated caregiver, combined with a tradition of constricted communication about emotional issues, may make adaptation to illness and loss very difficult. An example is an Irish-American family in which a daughter and her child had AIDS. As is traditional in Irish families, the mother was the sole caregiver and this father was isolated, spending most of his time away from home or at home alone or with one of the sons. When the previously addicted daughter and her child were diagnosed, the affect system in the family completely closed down. The mother and daughter were the only members who spoke about the illness and, then, only about the practical issues. The split between the men and the women in the family widened. A rigid oppressive silence about the illness created intense antagonism. The isolation of the family members from each other was such that no one recognized that the second son, silently watching television with his father, was habitually injecting heroin and also at risk for AIDS.

AIDS has a high affective overload and demands communication about the complex psychosocial issues associated with it. For an Irish or Anglo-Saxon family, in which processing feelings may not be part of the usual style of communication, silence may impede practical care. Mourning processes may be impeded by the unavailability of other affective interaction. In the Irish family described above, the parents were unable to communicate with each other in their grief over the deaths of their daughter and granddaughter. The mother's grief was incapacitating, the father's isolation worsened, and the son's use of drugs increased. Eventually, the mother defied the family code of silence and communicated her grief to an outsider, a family therapist. As a result, communication within the family increased and symptoms decreased. However, without such intervention, the lack of communication might have led to greater fragmentation of the family. Psychotherapeutic intervention helped the family to learn new communication patterns, to risk sharing their feelings about the loss of the two family members, and, in turn, to begin to heal.

When AIDS forces disclosure about one's personal life, and after a family code of silence has been broken and communication has been initiated, a family may discover a degree of strength and cohesion that they had not experienced previously. In one Irish family, the gay son had never disclosed his sexual orientation to any family member except the brother to whom he was closest. The family was deeply connected by a history of struggle and love but did not discuss issues which would hurt their mother, a proud traditional woman and single parent who had struggled hard for her children's considerable success. When her son decided to disclose that he was gay and had AIDS, he was amazed at his mother's compassion and acceptance. The family felt strengthened, despite the tragedy, by a new closeness and by increased interaction and communication. The mother found it helpful to discuss some of the issues about the development of sexual orientation and to explore the son's internalized homophobia and protectiveness of her. She was able to resolve her guilt and express her sadness that for so many years he had felt he needed to conceal from her something so central to his life.

Because AIDS rapidly is becoming a major health problem in many minority communities, health professionals need to understand the culture of those communities and become sensitized to the difficulties presented by differences in language. The complex illness pattern of AIDS, and the proliferation of medical protocols available, demand that families with infected members master complex medical information seldom presented in their language. For example, in one Latino family, the decision to go on a drug protocol, which had many risks, required reading a large amount of information about side effects and possible outcomes. Because a Spanish interpreter was not provided, communication with their physician was difficult. Their decision to turn down the protocol may have been wise, or it may have occurred because they did not understand that the possible side effects were not inevitable.

Clinicians need to be sensitive to the cultural differences between them and the patient and his/her family. Deference to these differences is necessary to forge a workable provider-patient-family alliance that can survive the stresses associated with AIDS. Disregard of these issues is a major cause of noncompliance and treatment failure and can lead families to wall themselves off from health providers and available community resources. For instance, it is customary in some Italian and Jewish families to describe physical symptoms freely and in detail. Individuals from other cultural backgrounds, such as Irish or Anglo-Saxon, tend to deny or conceal ailments. One can envision the potential for misunderstanding and tension that could develop between Italian or Jewish health providers working with Anglo-Saxon patients and their families. A mutually frustrating cycle of health providers pursuing a distancing family could develop. At minimum, dissatisfaction would result. At worst, the family would leave treatment and use the negative experience as a rationale to rigidify its alienation and isolation from adequate care.

Hospital social workers and others who provide care may be overwhelmed by the problems minority families face when dealing with AIDS. These families may make demands that can lead to burnout if the therapist or caregiver assumes too much responsibility for family and patient. Despite difficulties of language and culture, many of these families have shown great resourcefulness in

other situations in which they needed to negotiate political and social systems. A more effective role is for the therapist to serve as
consultant to the family and (a) to help family members take a long-
range view of their needs over the course of the illness; (b) to give
them the information needed to understand medical alternatives and
to negotiate the hospital system; and (c) to assist them in locating
appropriate services and support groups. The health information
groups developed by the National Coalition of People With AIDS
are effective models for the dissemination of medical information in
hospital settings. Such problem-solving and educational groups are
often more useful to persons with AIDS and their families than
traditional support and therapy groups.

Religion

To understand the impact of AIDS on families, the helper needs
to understand the religious heritage of the client family and the
meaning which has been attached to homosexuality, drug use, and
AIDS. A family with a member dying of AIDS may want religious
consolation as may the individual. Some denominations, however,
have been punitive toward persons with AIDS, seeing the disease as
God's punishment for a deviant lifestyle. The family may echo this
position and "blame the victim." For example, a person may wish
to reconcile with his church but not wish to disown his sexual identity, his lover, or his gay world. The family may be helped to locate
clergy or rabbis who will be understanding, nonjudgmental, and
willing to work with persons with AIDS and their families to approach the spiritual dimension of the illness. Members of a congregation can be a very important support system, assuming caregiving
functions as well as providing spiritual support. Acceptance by a
religious or spiritual community can do much to counter the attribu-
tion of sin and guilt often associated with the disease.

Socioeconomic Class

Families in poverty may not feel confident to fight for better care,
know when treatment is inadequate, or risk overriding a physician's
recommendation when it is not best for the family. Educated middle-class families are better able to deal with hospital systems, to

demand the kind of care needed, and to access current medical information. For example, it is not unusual for a middle-class gay man to be extremely knowledgeable about the medical protocols available to him as an AIDS patient and to understand standard medical practice. He may know, for instance, that following a bout of PCP he should be maintained against recurrence, and he is likely to protest if his doctor does not prescribe such treatment. A person living in poverty may be unaware of such information and be grateful for any care given by physicians.

Low-income communities may be more overt in their stigmatization of AIDS than middle-class communities, but it is not clear that they actually have greater prejudice against persons with AIDS. They have had less access to AIDS information, such as safer-sex workshops and contact with articulate members of groups for persons with AIDS. Rumors about contamination are rampant in low-income communities, but it is probable that educated middle-class persons quietly harbor the same fears. Among the less advantaged, children whose parents have AIDS are stigmatized in the schools, but is not clear that such children are better treated among the middle and upper classes. In fact, the presence of irrational and often unacknowledged fears among health-care workers supports the notion that these fears are rampant in the middle class.

Good social service intervention is essential to provide families, especially poor families, with basic information regarding employment, finances, housing, and medical issues. Volunteer organizations, such as Gay Men's Health Crisis, often provide excellent support services and may have more resources than hospital social service systems which typically serve the poor. Some people in poverty may be hesitant to enroll for services because such groups have been associated with homosexuality.

Middle-class families are more likely to have good insurance coverage to pay much of the enormous medical costs of AIDS. A poor family that has worked hard to get off the welfare rolls may be forced back onto welfare because of job loss or extended sick leave when a member develops AIDS. Some middle-class work systems have been amenable to maintaining the person with AIDS on the payroll throughout the course of the illness. People with lower job status frequently are not as fortunate. When the family can no longer afford the apartment they had when the person with AIDS was working or when the needs for home care can no longer be fulfilled in the overcrowded living space, housing becomes a problem. In urban centers, such as New York and San Francisco, there are almost no housing units for homeless families with a family member ill with AIDS, and some of these families are consigned to shelters. If a family member has to take in children of parents who have died of AIDS, it may be hard for them to find adequate housing. If they have children, women with AIDS often have difficulty finding shelter.

PSYCHOSOCIAL NEEDS OF POPULATIONS AT RISK

When identifying populations at risk for AIDS, there is the danger that persons not in these groups will see themselves as separate from the problem. In a few years, this may be less likely when more of the general population knows someone with AIDS and when the notion of "high-risk groups" has less meaning. For now, the impact of AIDS is disproportionately high in groups holding minority status. To date, the primary subpopulation at risk for AIDS and HIV seropositivity has been gay and bisexual men. However, the prevalence of HIV is growing rapidly in other populations and a high percentage of persons at risk are IV drug users. A small proportion of persons with AIDS were infected by blood products received prior to Spring, 1985, and, although their numbers are small, it is estimated that as many as 90% of the hemophiliac population may be seropositive (CDC, 1987). Sexual partners and children of IV drug users, bisexual men, and blood product recipients are rapidly growing subpopulations at risk, and the disease is moving into the non-high-risk heterosexual populations. These shifts pose new problems, present new patterns of response, and offer family professionals much uncharted territory.

Gay Men

The HIV epidemic impacts on gay men in numerous significant ways. Potential and actual infection affects their intimate relationships and their sexual lives, a diagnosis of AIDS raises unresolved issues with families of origin, community fear and misinformation amplify the classically pervasive discrimination against homosexuality, and a positive HIV antibody test stimulates latent guilt and internalized homophobia.

A therapist treating the gay population must be informed about and sensitive to the sexual mores of the gay community and to the dynamics of the male couple (e.g., see McWhirter & Mattison, 1984). Sex outside of a committed relationship has been seen by many gay men as a positive good and has been associated with sexual and gay liberation (Altman, 1982, 1987). However, the HIV epidemic has required a re-evaluation of this sexual practice. Many gay men do not want to return to what was considered homophobic sexual moralism or give up the sexual freedom which they have come to value, but they are aware that "unsafe" sex with multiple partners is dangerous and endangering.

Although it can be argued that the AIDS crisis actually creates better and more intimate relationships by encouraging monogamy for gay men, this bias in the therapy relationship may reify a secret fear that AIDS is indeed a punishment. Therapists must respect sexual values and behaviors which may be different than their own while emphasizing the necessity for sexual responsibility and commitment to safer-sex practices to protect self and others.

A key issue for therapists working with gay couples is the delicate nature of their relationship with their families of origin. Often a couple will be close to the family of one partner whereas the other partner's family does not know of their son's homosexuality. The diagnosis of AIDS forces a double "coming out," the simultaneous disclosure of a fatal illness and of homosexuality (Tiblier, 1987). Even if the family may be accepting of their son's disclosure, they may be unaccepting of the lover and this reaction may further stress the couple's relationship. Conflicts of loyalty may arise between a wish to be reunited with one's family of origin and a commitment to a lover. In some cases, the person with AIDS may decide not to disclose and, instead, to maintain a cut-off or distant relationship with his parents and siblings. This is likely to create special problems for the family and the partner at time of death. When illness is accompanied by a realization that reconciliation with family will never occur, there may be renewed anger and mourning for that loss.

Professionals must be careful not to impose their beliefs about the value of reconnecting with family of origin. One must be guided by the possible effects on the person who has been diagnosed, the lovers, and the larger family unit. Long-term damage can result from poor handling of this crisis period, and it requires considerable courage and determination for persons to counteract old attitudes and patterns of interaction. Families may react to "coming out" with initial rejection, and an individual with AIDS may be too vulnerable to face further censure and rejection by emotionally significant persons. However, when reconciliation can be managed, the benefits are considerable. *It is crucial to remember that any decision to seek family alliances must be made by the person with AIDS.*

The often slow process of reconciliation is begun usually by helping the individual identify family members who would be most likely to support him. The therapist must help the patient to anticipate ways to cope with the potential rejection and censure he may encounter and encourage him to develop and utilize alternative support networks as a buffer.

A major source of strength for gay men with AIDS is the community support system. The success of San Francisco's gay community in educating its members about prevention measures is reflected in the lowered rates of new infection. Self-help groups have empowered people with AIDS to take charge of their medical needs by providing current medical information, treatment alternatives, and a politically active and knowledgeable support network. Groups such as Gay Men's Health Crisis and Shanti have provided models of compassionate care which cut through the bureaucratic morass and are a source of gay pride and self-affirmation. Similar models must be developed for other populations infected with the disease.

IV Drug Users

The second most common HIV-infected population are IV drug users and their sexual partners. In large cities, these persons are located disproportionately in black and Latino communities.

Persons who inject heroin, cocaine, and amphetamines are at

high risk for AIDS because the drug-taking ritual often includes sharing needles and, hence, blood may be exchanged in the process. If users support themselves through prostitution, they are, in fact, in two high-risk categories. In minority communities, the majority of IV drug users are heterosexuals whose sexual contacts and children are, in turn, placed at risk for AIDS. In communities where serial relationships are common and there is a high incidence of addiction, there is a greater likelihood that a woman will have a sexual relationship with an IV drug user.

People who are addicted may be difficult to reach and hard to teach. Hence, it may be necessary to work directly with the family, who may be more easily available and who need information about the disease. Because drug users often have a high degree of contact with their families of origin, some form of family therapy should be considered when working with this population (see Stanton & Todd, 1982).

It has been common therapeutic policy to treat the drug user alone or in peer groups rather than with family members. This approach is based on the belief that "cure" involves separation from the childlike role usually taken with the family or spouse and the establishment of an independent life. However, because drug users may be elusive and secretly enmeshed with their families, what an addicted person says to the therapist about independence from family may be fictitious. Family behavior is often a powerful reinforcement of drug use and the person who uses drugs may be extremely sensitive to family cues. Frequently, attempts to change behavior are accompanied by family upheaval, which, in turn, may precipitate renewed drug use. Working with the spouse to modify sexual behavior and to give up the role of caretaker/enabler is often more productive than attempting to work with the user alone (see Stanton & Todd, 1982).

Recently diagnosed persons who are drug-dependent are likely to be in a state of terror and denial. They are apt to deal with AIDS with characteristic defenses (i.e., drugs, flight). By working through the spouse/partner or family of origin, the therapist reduces panicky isolation, draws the person with AIDS from the street community to which s/he may have fled upon diagnosis, and offers an alternative source of nurturance and care. If the individual remains isolated and is not brought into some kind of care, s/he is likely to put others at risk through continued sexual and drug practices. If intervention is successful and the drug user chooses to enter a therapeutic program, work with the family can be helpful to support attempts to change.

Because the family may have a history of tension, frustration, and failure with the addicted member, it is often difficult to engage them in therapy when that individual becomes HIV-infected. To the family who has spent years attempting to rescue the user from his habit, AIDS is the ultimate sign of failure. The family may well choose to deal with this sense of futility by distancing from the user or by making even more frantic attempts to rescue its addicted member. Because parents of drug users tend to blame their child's behavior on others (e.g., the "wrong" friends or the people who sell drugs on the streets), they often view persons outside the family as responsible for changing the behavior (e.g., courts, doctors, and therapists). This is likely to put additional pressure on the health-care team.

Women and AIDS

Women who use IV drugs or have heterosexual contact with IV drug users or bisexual men are at risk for AIDS. The occurrence of HIV infection in women is of special concern and infected mothers are the major source of infection for infants. Often a woman does not know she is infected until her baby is diagnosed with AIDS and, because the very fact of pregnancy activates and accelerates her own disease process, her death may occur prior to that of her child. Most women with AIDS are from minority populations living in poverty, and many mothers of children with AIDS live in single-parent households. Thus, to be ill with a debilitating disease adds the ultimate stressor to an already stressed situation.

The prevention of HIV infection presents particular problems for women. Because of their socialization into a passive gender role, many women find it hard to assert themselves sufficiently to ensure safer-sex practices. It is important to educate all women about their risk of sexually-acquired AIDS and to encourage risk-reducing behaviors. Women must be counseled to reduce their risk by insisting that their partners always use condoms during intercourse, especially if they or their lover may have multiple partners or use IV drugs. Women should be taught to utilize a diaphragm or sponge with the spermicide, Nonoxynol-9. All women whose behaviors or partners put them at risk of HIV infection should consider being tested for HIV antibodies before becoming pregnant or immediately upon learning that they are pregnant.

Hemophiliacs

The hemophiliac population is heavily at risk for AIDS and as many as 90% may be HIV-infected. Because many hemophiliacs are married, spouses and unborn children are also at risk. The current conversion rate of HIV-infected hemophiliacs to AIDS is somewhat below that of other populations, perhaps because their immune systems have been less compromised.

The therapist working with the hemophiliac population must be sensitive to the particular problems they face. Because the management of hemophilia has been achieved by carefully controlling much of their environment, infection with HIV may destroy hemophiliacs' fundamental trust in their ability to control their fate. The medical world upon whom they have relied is now known to have been mistaken about the safety of infusion as a method of bleed control. Official medical information in this country was unrealistically optimistic regarding the low risk of contamination from the blood supply. Throughout the medical career of the hemophiliac and his family, the medical system has played the role of trusted advisor, often saving the hemophiliac's life. Now, despite the sense of betrayal, the hemophiliac and his family are still inextricably tied to the very system which has failed them.

Because stress can bring on life-threatening bleeds, hemophiliacs have learned to keep tension, passion, and emotionality under careful control. Their parents have learned a similar style of emotional control, allowing them thus to preserve their child's life. By managing emergencies with as much calm as possible, they have assisted their child through painful and frightening medical procedures, schooled him to avoid physical danger, and agonized silently as he approached the risk-taking years of adolescence. The anger prompted by a diagnosis of HIV infection may be converted to despair, intense depression, and psychosomatic symptoms in a system forbidding direct emotional expression.

For the hemophiliac with AIDS, the diagnosis is often the first experience of being part of a socially stigmatized group. To the adolescent hemophiliac who has struggled to lead a normal life, AIDS now brings the label of abnormal and deviant (see Goffman, 1963). The hemophiliac with AIDS usually suffers this social stigmatization in isolation. Networks available to gay men or to IV drug users may seem alien to a person who has tried to melt into the "normal" middle-class community and not be seen as different. Wives of infected hemophiliacs, who accepted the traditional problems associated with hemophilia when they married, now are faced with new issues — the possibility of their own contamination and, perhaps, a future without children.

Hemophiliacs have been socialized to believe that by personal effort and mastery they can control their disease. Those who reach adulthood have learned to moderate emotions and to master physical limitations, pain, and disability. AIDS, a disease of intense uncertainty, apparently defying control, is a new experience to the hemophiliac. Because the hemophiliac is used to finding that personal effort leads to success, the terminal phase of AIDS may be accompanied by a profound sense of failure. The positive side is that these families can be excellent candidates for family therapy, and one can anticipate their cooperation and efforts to utilize the experience.

Persons Infected by Blood Transfusions

Persons who have been infected by blood transfusion are likely to be in fairly traditional heterosexual relationships. As with other groups, contamination fears and feelings of social stigma and isolation accompany diagnosis. Because blood transfusion infection is a random event, the family may create explanations which blame self or others in order to give some meaning to the illness. These may involve notions of guilt, sin, or punishment for imagined or actual past deeds. There may be a reaction similar to that observed in hemophiliacs of feeling betrayed by the medical system. This response could interfere with the family's seeking appropriate help.

An additional problem is the paucity of support groups specifically designed for women or men who have acquired HIV infection through transfusion.

HIV-Infected Children

As the disease spreads to women, the number of children with AIDS is increasing, especially among minorities. Hundreds of infected babies will be born each year, many of these in New York City. The majority of these babies will be born to women who are IV drug users or the sexual partners of users, and many are black or Latino. A smaller percentage of children and adolescents with AIDS are infected because of blood infusions prior to 1985. The number of adolescents with AIDS is low, perhaps because the incubation period is relatively long and those infected during adolescence show symptoms in their twenties.

If a mother is seropositive, there is probably a 50% chance that her baby also will be infected. Because the maternal antibody may be passively acquired in utero and may persist in the infant for up to 8 months or more, it is difficult to determine an accurate diagnosis of HIV-infection in newborns (see Cooper, 1988). Thus, issues of day care, immunizations, and treatment are difficult to resolve until true infectivity can be established, and the family may have to live for an extended period without a definitive diagnosis. At time of pregnancy, many infected women are asymptomatic and, hence, unaware of their infection. Thus, a woman may learn simultaneously that she and her infant are seropositive. Moreover, because pregnancy may compromise the immune system, the pregnant infected woman may move more quickly to full-blown AIDS and many die within several years after giving birth.

The psychosocial implications for families of pediatric AIDS are numerous (see Urwin, 1988). Among the more obvious are (a) secrecy resulting from shame and fear of social isolation; (b) issues in the couple system resulting from fears of contamination, need to change sexual patterns, guilt, and anger; (c) possible illness and death of two parents, leaving the children as orphans; (d) issues of medical treatment and child care for the infected child; (e) impact on the sibling system, which may experience fear and resentment;

and (f) issues related to death and bereavement as experienced by the entire family system.

When a baby has AIDS, the human service professional is often dealing with a dying system. Both parents are at risk and both may die. Siblings may be forced to take on responsibilities far beyond those appropriate for their age. If parents have not told the extended family, they too must keep the secret and may feel extraordinarily isolated. They may live with the fear that their parents may die but with little sense of external support. If they know a baby brother or sister has AIDS, they quickly learn that they and their family can be stigmatized by the community. The family professional must work to build extended family relationships so that the children can feel nurtured by other adults in addition to their parents and plans can be made for a future which may not include their parents.

Some hospitals have developed support groups for children who have siblings or parents with AIDS. However, because of the stigma attached to participation and because they prefer to comfort themselves with the fiction that "mommy will get better," it is often hard to engage children in these groups. Sometimes it is helpful to teach older family members how to help the children talk about these feelings.

Appropriate care for the HIV-infected child is difficult (see Cooper, 1988). There are potential hazards to standard immunizations with live vaccine, recurrent infections, and frequent and devastating instances of central nervous system infection. Although there has been no documentation of HIV transmission in schools, day care, or other such settings, and current CDC guidelines specify that school-age HIV-infected children can be included in the classroom, education of such children has been an emotionally charged topic. It is recommended that the decision be based on the general health of the child and on whether attendance would risk undue exposure to opportunistic infections. Many programs exclude seropositive children under 3 years of age from attending day care, thus creating further economic and supervision issues for the family.

Many babies who are born with AIDS remain in the hospital because their families cannot provide care. Social service policy usually is to seek adoptive or foster homes for these children, a policy which has its own attendant problems. The adoptive or foster parent often harbors fears of contamination from blood and fecal products, and there are complicated ethical questions regarding confidentiality of the infant's serostatus. In one case, adoptive parents of a baby with AIDS decided to tell no one — neither relatives, babysitters, nor day care workers. They had great concern that their families would learn of their secret and criticize them for the decision to adopt an infected child. Because the child played with nieces and nephews, there was a fear that their siblings would find out and be enraged. The secrecy surrounding their baby soon created a rigid boundary around the couple. Unable to talk to others about their concerns, all anxieties were kept within the couple system, causing mounting conflict.

Those who care for AIDS babies live with the knowledge that their baby will die. Hence, they must find strategies to keep going, often maintaining the belief that this baby will be the one child who recovers. Stress in the couple relationship can arise when one parent becomes despondent and fearful about the child's impending death and the other parent insists on optimism and denial. The high degree of psychological distress and the enormous amount of medical attention required for AIDS babies frequently bring couples or single parents to counseling. The complications for the family which surround pediatric AIDS are essentially unprecedented in medical history, and it requires exceptional skill to help families find the strength necessary to cope effectively (see Bluebond, 1978; U.S. Department of Health and Human Services, 1987; Walker, 1988).

Partners of HIV-Infected Persons

Partners face anticipatory grief and the eventual need to reorganize their own lives without the other. They face the tasks of caregiving, working with hospital systems and other professionals, and fears about their own futures. There is tremendous anxiety attached to further sexual activity within the relationship and, in turn, even expression of affection may be curtailed. Unmarried partners may receive pressure from their own relatives to leave the relationship or the infected individual may be encouraged to return to the family of origin for care.

A major issue for all partners is whether or not to be tested. The

decision is complicated and personal, involving considerable interpersonal risk. Partners fear that finding out they are positive will
overwhelm their ability to care for an ill partner or even to remain in
the relationship. As one wife said, "If I find I am negative I will
wonder if I should leave before I am infected. If I find that I am
positive, I will hate him forever." Professionals must keep in mind
that the smaller the relationship arena, the more intense the pressure
on that system. Whenever possible, they should encourage broad-
ening that arena to include other family, friends, professionals, and
volunteers.

BIOPSYCHOSOCIAL STAGES ASSOCIATED WITH THE MEDICAL COURSE OF AIDS

To look at AIDS through a biopsychosocial lens leads to two
separate but interrelated perspectives. First, one can describe the
psychosocial issues associated with the illness at each of the medical stages from wellness to death, including (a) the "worried well,"
(b) report of HIV-seropositivity, (c) diagnosis of ARC, (d) diagnosis of AIDS, (e) death and bereavement, and (f) family reorganization. Second, all chronic and life-threatening illnesses can be described in terms of the following time phases (see Rolland, 1984,
1987a): (a) crisis, (b) chronic, and (c) terminal. Each phase has its
own developmental tasks and requires different coping and adaptation skills from the family. Each of the biopsychosocial stages will
be discussed separately with its related psychosocial issues. Attention then will be given to the psychosocial developmental tasks associated with the crisis, chronic, and terminal stages of HIV-infection. Although there will be some overlap in the issues discussed, it
is helpful to consider them from the two perspectives of stage and
time.

Biopsychosocial Stages

The "Worried Well"

There is a growing population of persons, often referred to as the
"worried well," who fear that past experiences have exposed them
to the HIV virus. This group is composed predominately of (a) per-

sons who fear exposure from past experimentation with IV drugs or sexual involvement with partners in high-risk categories, and (b) health-care workers, such as medical residents, nurses, paramedics, and laboratory technicians. Because the fear of AIDS is so prevalent, people who have only a single sexual encounter with someone thought to be at risk may become obsessed with anxiety, depression, or rage. Each physical symptom seems to confirm the fears of the "worried well." Counseling may be useful to help persons in this category make decisions about whether to be tested for possible HIV seropositivity.

The decision to test is a complicated one. With the social stigma attached to AIDS, many fear that testing will jeopardize their civil liberties. Positive diagnosis may result in increased psychiatric and psychosomatic symptoms, including anxiety, depression, inhibition of sexual desire, and symptoms mimicking ARC (e.g., headaches, fevers, coughs, and diarrhea). The family and relationship systems will be thrown into severe stress at the same time that diagnosis places its own stresses on the individual.

On rare occasions, a test may yield "false positive" results, requiring repeated testing to ascertain whether the results are accurate. Because of the lag between infection and the development of antibodies, it is also possible to receive a "false negative" result. Knowing this, some "worried well" find it difficult to be reassured by a negative result and so demand multiple testings.

Seropositivity

Seropositivity is a dividing line between normal life and life at risk for fatal illness. Even medically asymptomatic persons who are seropositive must accept that they have a high probability of developing AIDS and of premature death.

Seropositivity is the beginning of the crisis phase of the illness, when the person starts to experience a shift in identity from healthy to ill and from normal to stigmatized. The individual has become someone whose body is inhabited by a virus associated in the public mind with a wide range of negative connotations — sinful, deviant, poisonous, and contaminated. Though asymptomatic, the seropositive person must develop coping mechanisms to deal with powerful

Damoclean fears. Some deal with this acute anxiety by actually denying the possibility of becoming ill.

For those who are single, painful decisions must be made about what to reveal in any subsequent sexual relationships. For the person who has been in a long-term relationship such as marriage or long-term cohabitation, there are crucial issues about disclosure to the partner, accompanied by fears that the partner will choose to leave the relationship. In many cases, a revelation of seropositivity is accompanied by a revelation of bisexuality, drug involvement, or extramarital affairs about which the partner may not have previously known, at least not consciously. As a result, issues related to betrayal can become a major theme as the couple seeks to integrate and to resolve emotions aroused by the new information and to make decisions about the future.

In a marriage where the infected partner has been drug-addicted, the well spouse may have spent years hoping to rescue the partner from self-destruction only to find that even his/her own life is now at risk. It is normal to feel bitter, impotent, and scared, and, at this point, many decide finally to leave the relationship. Because the seropositive person may sense this possibility, s/he may choose not to reveal the seropositivity and even to continue unprotected sex.

The response to testing is not always so bleak. Many gay men who have tested HIV-positive have helped one another treat the diagnosis as a challenge. In such a case, seropositivity can change sexual relationships for the better, increasing intimacy and encouraging persons to be more open, honest, and caring about their partners. Safer-sex workshops typically emphasize the potential for warmth and intimacy that is possible in sex when it is protective and loving of the partner.

Nevertheless, anyone who is diagnosed as seropositive must go through a period of mourning for the loss of identity as a healthy person and for the necessary changes in one's sexual life. From now on, each new sexual encounter will be problematic and may involve uncomfortable questioning and possible rejection if one is honest about one's serostatus.

Parents who test seropositive may fear for the lives of recently born children who also may have to be tested. If they have older children, they ponder the future of these children and how long they will have to parent them. They wonder about the wisdom of sharing their test results with the children or whether this will only serve to create unnecessary anxiety and potential ostracism. Children may sense their parents' worry, which heightens their own insecurity.

The period of accepting seropositivity is likely to be stormy for the couple relationship. There may be difficult questions like, "What was the nature of our relationship that we did not know each other well enough to share what was going on outside of our relationship?" and accusations like, "You have destroyed my life. No one will ever want me again now that they know you are infected." Couples will question whether they should stay together. A partner of a seropositive person who tests negative may decide s/he does not wish to risk further intimate interaction, or the seropositive individual may, out of feelings of guilt, shame, and protectiveness, seek to push the well partner out of the relationship.

The diagnosis of seropositivity hangs like a Damoclean sword over the infected person, the couple, and the family. From now on, they will always be on guard for further signs of infection and may become super-reactive to physical symptoms (see Callen, 1987). Diarrhea may be seen as the beginning of ARC, a cold the beginning of Pneumocystis. Many people become fanatical about revising their lifestyle — exercising, giving up cigarettes and alcohol, pursuing vitamin and nutritional therapy, and initiating meditation and yoga. Others deny their diagnosis, perhaps even increasing drug use and high-risk sex. The latter may be particularly true of the IV drug user population.

In a couple where one person is seropositive and the other is not, each partner may have a different time frame for life. The seropositive partner may want to focus on day-to-day issues, because planning ahead bears a shadow of illness and death. The seronegative partner may want life to seem normal and insist on planning for the future. This discrepancy in goals, with one person's life foreshortened and the other able to contemplate a normal lifespan, may push the couple out of synchronicity.

The fact that individuals are likely to become HIV-infected at an early stage in the lifecycle has important implications. A young man of 25, now drug free after an adolescent phase of drug abuse, suddenly finds that such normal life goals as marriage and children are closed to him. The life decisions he must now make are distinctly different than if he were to have become ill at a later stage in life when he had accomplished more of his life goals.

Seropositivity may result, for some, in a life of more conscious meaning. When an individual faces the possibility that s/he may have a fatal illness, unsatisfactory career choices may be thrown aside for new paths promising more fulfillment. Motivated to reevaluate life, persons may come to a new and deeper understanding of themselves and of their partners and families, and find ways to ensure that the life that remains will be well spent. It is not unusual in therapy to hear, "Now that I know I am at risk, I have begun to value my life in a new way and to do those things which I really want to do," or "Why did it take this to make me realize how much I love you!"

ARC Diagnosis

With the diagnosis of an AIDS Related Condition (ARC), the person moves from a world of chronic illness without medical symptoms to chronic illness with symptoms. These may include central nervous system deterioration, memory loss, failure of coordination, diarrhea, and extreme fatigue. Physical symptoms reactivate the threat of dying. Day-to-day debilitation may affect one's ability to work, and more and more sick days may be taken. Financial stability is threatened. There is a fear of job loss as employers question the number of missed workdays. In some states, it is illegal to dismiss a person from employment because of ARC or AIDS, but other reasons may be found for eventual termination. With loss of employment, one may also lose medical insurance.

Seropositivity was an invisible secret. Now secrecy must be kept in the face of visible physical symptoms. If the person with ARC begins to show weight loss, people begin to notice and to inquire. As the person becomes ill, decisions must be made about whether to inform friends and relatives. At some point, the fear of disclosure may be outweighed by the need to receive care. Whereas before it was only necessary to inform one's sexual partners, now one must decide when and how to disclose to children, parents, and friends. When the family network, in whatever form it exists, begins to rally in support of an individual with a chronic illness, the illness rapidly will become public.

It will not be easy for the individual or for his/her family to reorganize to meet the new demands. ARC may bring with it incapacitating symptoms ranging from reduced energy levels to specific cognitive or motor impairments. The person with ARC may be unwilling to yield previous roles and may resist caregiving. It will be important for the family to learn the rhythm of impairment, neither robbing the individual prematurely nor denying the incapacitation. Some families tend to distance themselves from a member who is terminally ill. Some have viewed the gay lifestyle as a conscious rebellion against family norms or have struggled with the individual's destructive use of drugs. These families may have difficulty trusting that the infected individual will now do what is necessary to protect them from contamination.

Although there is a medical distinction between ARC and AIDS, the ill person and the family may find the two indistinguishable. Physicians may offer reassurance that survival is longer with ARC, but many patients know enough to fear the conversion to AIDS and to realize that their lives are seriously shortened. Moreover, even though the person with ARC begins to feel general debilitation, the illness is severe, and life is perhaps threatened, ARC does not qualify one for the same financial disability benefits as AIDS.

AIDS Diagnosis

The course of AIDS is idiosyncratic, although, ultimately, it progresses to a terminal phase. If it begins with a life-threatening episode, such as Pneumocystis pneumonia, and if not successfully treated, AIDS can result in death in a matter of days. For some, there may be a protracted quiescent period, lasting for several years, punctuated only by episodic medical crises. Each type of course (progressive, constant, or relapsing/episodic) will make different psychosocial demands on the family (see Rolland, 1984, 1987a).

The progressive course of AIDS means that the family faces a continually symptomatic member whose illness acts in a stepwise or gradually debilitating manner. Although new treatment protocols, such as AZT, may provide longer periods of relative wellness, AIDS is a progressive illness with minimal asymptomatic periods. Continual adaptation and role change are required of everyone involved. Increasing strain on family caretakers is caused by both the risks of exhaustion and the accumulation of new caretaking tasks. Family adaptability is at a premium (see Helmquist, 1984).

For a time, the illness usually assumes a relapsing/episodic course, in which baseline symptoms and stable periods of varying length alternate with periods of medical crisis. The family can attempt to carry on its "normal" routine, but the specter of crisis continually looms. This episodic course demands that the family remain on-call, ready to form a crisis structure whenever necessary. The frequency of shifts from crisis to noncrisis, and the ongoing uncertainty of when a medical and perhaps life-threatening crisis will occur, puts considerable strain on caregivers. The disparity between periods of quiescence and periods of crisis and exacerbation may be particularly taxing.

The person with AIDS may have as long as 5 years or more to live or may be dead within a month of the first major infection leading to diagnosis. Several opportunistic infections may be present simultaneously or sequentially and may require hospitalization. Between these acute illnesses, there may be long periods of relatively good health. Although fatigue, weight loss, and diarrhea may accompany less acute phases, these symptoms may not be severe enough to prevent the individual from engaging in normal activities. At other times, he or she may feel increasingly debilitated. Death may come suddenly, when the patient appears to be in relatively good health, or there may be a progressive deterioration over time, possibly with central nervous system involvement and mental deterioration. The patient may be homebound for a long period during which there is increasing disorientation, disturbance, and loss of control over bodily functions (see Schoen, 1986). Because there is no single predictable course of the illness, families must be able to move back and forth between two modes of operation — one which is primarily focused on care and one which allows the patient to resume some of the normal functioning essential to psychological well-being.

Because the symptoms of AIDS are so varied and so complex,

the family must be vigilant for signs of onset of a new medical emergency, and caregivers may be the first to identify an opportunistic infection. Often it is hard for family members to help the person with AIDS determine when medical intervention is needed. If one of the first signs of new infection is mental deterioration, it may be difficult to distinguish between a biological event and a psychological state, and the family may become divided in their interpretation. The following examples illustrate this point.

In one case of a gay man with undiagnosed AIDS dementia, the family attributed his depression and apathy to his relationship with his lover whom they detested. The lover believed that the behavior manifested serious organic change. Early neurological tests were inconclusive, but later testing, at the lover's insistence, confirmed an organic process.

Another case involved a man who had decided, with the support of other family members, to tell his mother about both his homosexuality and his diagnosis. She surprised him by her acceptance, and, although his coming-out was traumatic, he found it a relief. The day after the disclosure the patient experienced difficulty breathing. Because this man had a reputation for hysterical symptoms, the family thought he was experiencing anxiety about his mother's response. In fact, he was showing early signs of a new round of Pneumocystis pneumonia. Whether stress following events like disclosure can make a patient more susceptible to infection, and in what ways, is not fully understood. In any event, it seems important that the family professional help patients and families find ways of reducing stress and of using potentially stressful events, such as disclosure, as opportunities to provide emotional support for one another (see Helmquist, 1984).

It is important to understand ways in which illness may be utilized dysfunctionally in ongoing family struggles. The person with AIDS may derive enormous secondary gains from the diagnosis and may be shrewd at manipulating family beliefs and guilt to gain power over other family members. Not all persons with AIDS and their families function well and the illness sometimes strikes families who require treatment by a skilled psychotherapist (see Beavers, 1982).

On the one hand, because AIDS is a fatal illness, the life of the patient and the family may be colored by anticipatory grief and pervasive hopelessness. On the other hand, some persons are able to adopt an attitude of hopefulness in the face of their illness (see Hughes & O'Neil, 1987). If the family does not adopt an attitude of optimism, the patient's morale may be negatively affected. People appear to do better when they are optimistic and when they can experience some control over decision making about their illness. Families can best facilitate patient functioning by providing care during the helpless periods of acute illness and by pulling back during remission to allow the patient to recover physical and mental independence.

Because so little is known about how to treat AIDS, families have to weigh carefully the advisability of drug protocols which have both benefits and negative side effects. AZT, for example, may begin to destroy bone marrow and make biweekly transfusions necessary. A family which initially encouraged this treatment may experience intense emotional confusion when faced with these negative consequences.

Finally, families have to deal with the social stigma still associated with the disease. As the infection progresses and increased treatment and care are necessary, it will be increasingly difficult to conceal the reality from the rest of the world. As others learn and react, the family is in danger of stigmatization by the community within which it resides (Tiblier, 1987).

Bereavement and Reorganization

Bereavement issues differ for different populations, but the common element is that people with AIDS tend to be young and their death is out of phase with the expected lifecycle. Children die before parents, parents die leaving young children, and several persons in the same family network may die in the same time period. In the late 20th century in the U.S. we are not accustomed to handling losses on such a large scale. Groups for survivors may prove helpful as family members, friends, and lovers attempt to resume normal living.

For the male couple, the loss of a partner to AIDS elicits a particularly complex set of responses and issues. In many cases, the dead lover becomes idealized during the terminal phases of his illness and after death. Out of intense feelings of love and grief, lovers may give up safer-sex practices and hope for mutual death. Because of the intense loneliness and isolation which can ensue after the death of a gay partner with AIDS, thoughts of suicide are not unusual. Feelings of guilt may be experienced by the individual who chose not to stay with his partner through the process of dying. Reorganization after death will have an entirely different meaning for the gay man who is himself seropositive and who fears that he too will die of AIDS in a few years. Out of his own intense grief, he may be tempted to enter too quickly into a new relationship, perhaps even concealing his seropositivity from his new partner (see Gilbert, 1988).

If the dead person was addicted, the family may have great difficulty in letting go. In some cases, the drug user's death is tied emotionally to a death in a previous generation. When the addict becomes terminally ill with AIDS the family may experience intense failure and a reawakening of the unresolved mourning issues connected with earlier losses. Some handle these issues by cutting off from their addicted member, whereas others become involved in rescue attempts that reach beyond the grave. Lawsuits against hospital staff for failing to save the individual are sometimes ways of keeping the person "alive." Surviving spouses of persons who were addicted may themselves be HIV-positive and have one or more children with AIDS. As they mourn the death of the spouse, they also are experiencing anger and helplessness regarding the likely death of other family members. Thus, the mourning becomes a mourning for their own curtailed life as well as that of others (see Walker, 1987).

When parents die of AIDS, their children are often bewildered by the surrounding secrecy and isolation. It is hard to grieve when one cannot discuss openly the cause of death. At the death of the parent, the sibling system may be split up and, thus, separation from the parent by death is made worse by separation also from brothers and sisters. During the terminal phase of the parent's illness, the siblings may have grown exceptionally close to one another, with the older ones caring for the younger. With separation, the support they have built for each other disappears. It is important that this sort of family breakup be avoided and that, when possible, a new family form be organized around the survivors.

Parents of adult children who die of AIDS will have conflicting emotions about a child who dies before them (see Shanfield et al., 1984, for related discussion). Often they feel a degree of guilt and inadequacy that they were not able to protect their child from a lifestyle that was apparently responsible for his/her death. Sometimes there is anger at a society which did not do a better job of educating about prevention or anger at themselves for whatever recrimination or discrimination they may have shown. Parents of gay persons have been helpful in providing support for other parents who otherwise might feel extraordinarily isolated (see, e.g., efforts by Visiting Nurses and Hospice of San Francisco to establish a network of parents of persons diagnosed with AIDS).

Sometimes, during the course of the illness, as with other life-threatening or terminal illnesses, adult children who have been cut off from their parents and adult siblings are reconciled. Often this is at the motivation and instigation of the person who is ill. As discussed above, reconciliation is not always easy and often requires the assistance of a skilled systems therapist who can help the entire system reconnect in the most appropriate manner and time frame. Sometimes a family has its own intuitive sense of how best to restore the system, so that all that is required of the therapist is a healthy respect for the good work they are doing on their own.

Psychosocial Time Phases of AIDS

Crisis

The crisis phase includes the initial period of readjustment and coping after the confirmation of seropositivity, ARC, or AIDS. During this period there are a number of key tasks for the infected person and his/her family (see Moos, 1984, for description of universal illness-related tasks): (a) learning to deal with AIDS-related symptoms (e.g., diarrhea, memory impairment, and fatigue); (b) learning to interact with the hospital environment and any AIDS-related medical treatments; and (c) establishing and maintaining workable relationships with the health-care team. In addition, there are critical tasks of a more general, existential nature (see Rolland, 1987a) which the family needs to accomplish: (a) explain the occurrence of AIDS in a way that maximizes a sense of mastery and competency; (b) grieve for the loss of the pre-illness family identity; (c) move toward acceptance of permanent change while maintaining a sense of continuity between past and future; (d) pull together to undergo short-term crisis reorganization; and (e) develop a family flexibility regarding future goals consistent with the inevitable uncertainty.

The crisis phase provides the initial framing of the illness, as the ill person and his/her family deal with the shocking event of diagnosis with its many medical, psychological, and relationship ramifications. A period of intense vulnerability precedes the development of ways of adapting to the illness. For this reason, health providers need to be particularly sensitive during this phase to the enormous positive and negative impact they can have on a vulnerable family. The first acute illness confronts the patient with pain and physical impairment, and the family is confronted with what may seem like an overnight change in the individual from healthy to ill. There is a need to deal simultaneously with the shock of the AIDS diagnosis and with the awareness of the loss of present and future health.

Acute infections may result in debilitation and weakness. Recovery may take as long as 2 or 3 months, and individuals may continue to feel tired, have episodic diarrhea, and lose weight. Persons with AIDS report that their bodies feel significantly different after the first round of acute illness. They can no longer carry out tasks with customary ease. The daily routine changes in that medication now becomes a major part of life. They become glued to the medical system, anxiously awaiting the latest red cell or T-cell count. They learn to identify the earliest signs of opportunistic infections, become aware of new protocols, and study the pros and cons of new drugs. The family learns, also, to monitor any physical or psychiatric changes which might herald such illnesses as toxoplasmosis or AIDS dementia.

A major task for the patient and the family is learning to deal with the hospital environment. The first hospitalization may be a highly unpleasant experience for the patient, who begins, as a consequence of staff treatment, to perceive himself as contaminated. Watching gloved and masked caregivers perform routine procedures, the person realizes that s/he is no longer ''normal.'' One is now viewed as fearsome, a person who can contaminate and kill. Despite any efforts of ombudsmen, the patient senses the fear of the hospital workers. As the family visits and for the first time sees the warnings of "infectious illness" on the door, they too may have a dramatic experience of viewing their family member as contagious. Family members may react in various ways—isolating the person with AIDS, banding together in protective outrage, arguing over the meaning of the illness, or "rolling up their sleeves" and beginning to make constructive plans.

Hospitals which serve as AIDS centers are flooded with patients and have overworked staff unable to give extra services. They often have difficulty attracting staff and residents. These conditions make it difficult for patients and health-care teams to establish the caring medical team/patient relationships so necessary to treating this complex disease. Even the best of doctors often do not have time to discuss symptoms directly with their patients and, therefore, turn over routine discussions to assistants. Because AIDS is complex, dangerous, and of uncertain course, some patients feel intensely dependent on the primary care of physicians. In the gay community, the problem of physician unavailability has often had the positive effect of creating medical-information self-help groups which encourage patients to become experts on the illness. Some groups even import controversial new drugs and establish protocols. These information channels are not readily accessible to minority family members, who constitute the newest high-risk group and who are frequently homophobic. Such families must absorb and integrate complex medical information but with less community help and with too few people who can interpret the information, particularly if they are not English-speaking.

Other developmental tasks are of a more existential nature. A major task during the beginning phase of any chronic illness is that the family interpret the experience in a way which allows them to preserve the sense of competency and self-esteem essential to coping and adaptation. This task is more difficult with AIDS because of the negative cultural meanings attributed to the illness—"the new plague," punishment for "deviant" behavior, "God's way of scourging an immoral society." These beliefs are buttressed by the fact that the source of infection, in many cases, is behavior considered immoral by the larger culture. The subgroups initially most attacked by this illness are already the most stigmatized — gays, minorities, prisoners, and immigrants. Some families are able to work through their initial self-deprecatory thoughts to arrive at a more calm and rational attitude. AIDS may burn away that which is trivial and replace surface relationships with ones that are more honest and searching.

It is essential to learn from family members what meanings they attach to illness and death and, in particular, to AIDS and to help them explore alternative interpretations. Although people with AIDS, their partners, and their families may discover meanings that redeem the experience, the process of doing so is likely to be painful and wrenching. At times, the AIDS process may threaten or even tear apart the fragile fabric of a family system or partnership.

Family identity following an AIDS diagnosis will never be the same and the family must start to mourn that loss. If the person with AIDS is a parent, there is a high chance that the partner and even the children may be infected. Because both "family executives" may die, leaving the children unparented, reorganization of the nuclear family to include members of the extended family/kin system often must begin at the point of diagnosis. This incorporation of other family members may be a difficult procedure if there are residual angers, feuds, and jealousies. The powerful stigma of AIDS creates a new family structure, with new coalitions and new boundaries. Family boundaries may become more rigid as the family interfaces with community systems and learns to keep its own counsel out of fear of being stigmatized at school, at work, or by friends. Yet boundaries between the family and the medical system need to become more permeable, rather than less, in order for the family system to absorb the numerous health-care workers and human-service personnel.

Normal executive functions of the family may be delegated to health-care workers, particularly if the head of the family is the person with AIDS. An increasing number of low-income women, many of them single parents, are affected by the illness. In some cases, as various family members step in to assume the functions left vacant by the ill person, rivalries occur between health-care workers and family members or between different factions in the family. In other cases, the health-care worker may be absorbed into the family. Determining and maintaining appropriate degrees of distance and closeness to the client family is often difficult.

Families with AIDS must find ways of maintaining a sense of continuity with past history. This may be especially hard when the family feels lodged in a painful present, anticipating a frightful future. Remembrance of past experience may serve only to increase the anguish of present reality, bringing to the surface further feelings of guilt, failure, and betrayal.

Many families go through extended periods of self-examination and criticism before they can accept the illness. Often they agonize over their failure to protect one another from the lifestyles causing the illness. A prior history of failed rescue attempts, even at a different generational level, and unresolved guilt over the past may exacerbate present pain. A successful handling of the illness and family matters in the present can go a long way to alleviate this distress.

Families need to undergo short-term crisis reorganization as well as to develop enough flexibility to deal with the uncertainties that lie ahead. Given the unpredictable course of AIDS and the episodic nature of the illness, the task of short-term reorganization is particularly difficult. For example, if a bisexual man's diagnosis is the first open acknowledgement of his sexual orientation, his wife may or may not wish to continue the relationship. Her uncertainty about her willingness to remain involved will drastically impair the family's ability to organize for caregiving. This phase of working through issues may take several months, a long time when dealing with an illness which has a relatively short lifespan. In most life-threatening illnesses, there is far less possibility that a relationship will break up upon diagnosis of the illness.

Chronic Phase

The chronic phase of AIDS, whether long or short, follows the initial adjustment period and precedes the terminal phase. With a fatal illness like AIDS, where hope for resuming a "normal" family life can only be realized after the death of the patient, this period is often a time of "living in limbo." Families often assume an attitude called "day-to-day living with AIDS." By this stage of the illness, the patient and family often have come to grips psychologically and/or organizationally with the permanent changes presented by AIDS and have devised an ongoing modus operandi. The ability of the family to maintain a semblance of a normal life under these abnormal circumstances is a key task of this period.

Another crucial task of this phase is the development of healthy autonomy for all family members in the face of a contradictory pull toward mutual dependency and caregiving. The family system must adapt itself to an illness in which part of the time the person with AIDS will be hospitalized with life-threatening illness, and part of the time he or she may be feeling relatively well and able to return to work and to resume the normal family role. During the chronic phase, the family must be prepared to deal with mental impairment as well as gradual loss of body function. In some instances, there will be central nervous system deterioration and dementia which may not require hospitalization but necessitates that someone remain at home with the patient. Sometimes children are thrust into this care role. It may be immensely disturbing for children to witness a parent slowly dying and, perhaps, unable to speak coherently or at all. With home care increasingly the norm with AIDS, it will be important to help children deal with the resulting stress.

Prior to the terminal phase, family members may be unable to think about preparation for death. While there is still life, many families wish to entertain hope and, in doing so, refuse to deal with the finality of the person's illness. In other cases, the family begins to wish for the death but feels guilty about such thoughts. Families respond with a range of emotions to the stresses of chronic illness and need help to sort these out as they arise.

Terminal Phase

The terminal phase of AIDS begins when the inevitability of death becomes apparent and is predominant in family thinking. For some, it ends with the death of the person with AIDS. For others who are at risk for the disease themselves, it continues into the perhaps distant future.

An important developmental task of the terminal phase is for the family as a unit, and for each of its members, to know that they have done what they could to help maintain contact with, and to care for, the person who is dying. It is also important to help members of the family network talk about issues related to dying. What constitutes sufficient contact and care or adequate communication will vary greatly among families and among different cultural/ethnic groups. Some may need help in making explicit what they define as adequate care. Will they feel they have done enough if they have been able to provide compassionate care or only if they have been able to save the family member from death? Often families, or individual members, are *driven* to save the person who is ill. Paradoxically, a family's efforts to continue life can result in the dying person experiencing guilt for letting them down.

Family clinicians should assess the range of caregivers available within the family or intimate network. Certain members, especially children and adolescents, may deny their own needs for nurturance out of loyalty to a parent who is involved in primary caregiving. The caregiver, in an impossible overload situation, may indirectly express a wish for this kind of loyalty by stating admiration for their children's ability to "take care of themselves." Some caregivers may jealously guard the caretaking role, shutting out other family members who could be helpful and who could benefit by closer contact with the patient and with the dying process. All of these issues can have far-reaching, long-term implications for surviving family members and for the family unit.

The terminal phase of AIDS may be acute or protracted. If the final illness is acute, death will probably take place in the hospital. However, with the development of newer medications, many people live longer and die in other facilities or at home, gradually wasting away and often becoming noncommunicative and incontinent (see Schoen, 1986).

In the terminal phase, the dying person and the family may be out of sync with regard to their acceptance of death. This is particularly common in addictive families where the family has been involved in a rescue operation for many years. The rescue efforts may go on even at the death bed, with the family still trying to find new medications or procedures to postpone death. The dying person, on the other hand, may have already accepted the inevitability of death and wish to share feelings about this with other family members who may refuse to listen. One patient begged hospital staff to get the family therapist to help the family accept her acceptance of death. The family was unable to do so and continued to believe that the patient would recover. The patient was forced to remain in her accustomed role as "parents' protector," needing to reassure them at a time when she needed reassurance and comfort in her dying process.

During the terminal phase, decision making regarding where the person will die and the extent to which medical efforts will be made to extend life requires a family health-care team that respects the family's basic belief system (see Rolland, 1987b). The attitudes and behaviors of the medical team can have a major influence in either facilitating or hindering the family's efforts to deal with death. A medical team that maintains heroic efforts to prolong the terminal phase of an illness can convey confusing messages, and the family may find it difficult to interpret these continued lifesaving efforts. Is there really hope? Should the family redouble their faith in and support of further medical intervention? Do the physicians feel bound to exhaust all technical possibilities at their disposal, regardless of the odds of success? Are physicians committed to this course for ethical reasons (the "leave no stone unturned" philosophy) or because of fears concerning legal liability? Is the medical team having its own difficulties letting go emotionally, perhaps because of their own emotional attachment to the patient or their personal history with similar experiences?

Medical and mental health professionals' strong attachments to certain patients can be fueled by unresolved losses in their own lives. Sometimes health-care professionals and institutions collude in a pervasive societal wish to deny death as a natural process beyond technological control (Becker, 1973). Endless treatment can represent the medical team's inability to separate a general value regarding promoting life from the reality of what would in fact be best for a given patient. Professionals need to examine closely their motives for treatments geared toward cure rather than palliation, particularly when a patient may be entering the terminal phase. The decision to use every means to prolong life needs to be made with careful attention to the patient's wishes and the degree of consensus within the family regarding the preferred course of action.

During the terminal phase, the counselor will want to help the family, in whatever form it exists, to begin to plan for the future. Clearly the time to do this is when the patient is still active and can identify some of his or her wishes regarding the future. Sometimes, however, when the counselor wishes to raise these issues, patients are in denial and wish to believe that they will recover and resume taking responsibility for their families. Such people may not be willing to settle issues involving custody or property distribution. When the patient has been the sole caretaker of the children, and in order to avoid legal disputes after death, some effort should be made to plan early for the care of the children after death. Many human service workers become involved with immediate needs and do not think about long-range planning. As a result, after the death of one parent, the family may be thrust into family court to deal with litigation over where the children should be and with whom.

Another issue during the terminal phase is the family reorganization required to ensure that the children are not subject to neglect. While a parent is slowly dying at home, the children may be living with only a mother and a visiting home health-care attendant whose job does not include childcare. Relatives who come to visit the family may not wish to move the children because of fear of destroying the mother's remaining attachment to life and because the children do not want to leave. This lingering situation can go on for months or even a year. During this time the doctors may be trying a series of medical protocols to save the life of a patient who has already suffered neurological impairment. Unfortunately, in the attempt to save the patient, little thought may be given to the needs of the larger family system.

As a function of the above stress, the children, burdened by worries they cannot assimilate, may become symptomatic. In one family, the child was diagnosed as school phobic. The mother who had AIDS had not been designated as sufficiently ill to require a home-care attendant. A family interview established that the mother was without friends or other family members to support her and that a more plausible explanation for the child's school phobia was his refusal to leave his mother. It was clear that the child stayed at home to be with his ill mother during the day when her boyfriend had to go to work. To cover his real mission, he told his mother he was afraid to go to school because his classmates knew that she had AIDS. He was responding sensitively to her fear that she would die alone.

During the terminal phase of AIDS, family and friendship networks may need help in preparing for the death of the patient and in instructing their doctors to discontinue medical procedures. It may be necessary to arrange psychosocial support for the dying process, for example, a compassionate friend or a spiritual leader who can be with the family around the sick bed. If loved ones can be at peace about and available during the death process, the patient, in turn, may be comforted.

LONG-TERM AND MULTI-GENERATIONAL IMPLICATIONS

Murray Bowen, a pioneer family systems theorist, has hypothesized an "emotional shock wave" that follows the death of a significant family member (Bowen, 1987). Driven by anxiety, it moves throughout the family system impacting many persons in that system, even those who may have been relatively uninvolved with the deceased. Therapists who work in the Bowen tradition believe that the family which resists emotional cutoffs, or works to mend them, may experience fewer emotional or physical problems in future generations. Whatever their theoretical orientation, most family professionals agree that the family which rallies around the person with AIDS, expands its resources, and develops calm and open relationships will reap benefits for the entire present and future family system. It is with this goal in mind that we seek to develop clinical methods which may promote maximum emotional healing for all families stricken with AIDS.

In the years to come, it is likely that each of us will know or love someone with AIDS. Once this happens, familiar stereotypes such as "high-risk groups" will assume less importance. The question will then be: How best can our society provide compassionate and effective medical and mental health care, cover the enormous financial and emotional costs of AIDS, help families find the internal resources necessary to grow through the grief of infection and terminal illness, and create a safer and more humane environment for us all?

REFERENCES

Altman, D. (1987). *AIDS in the mind of America*. New York: Doubleday/Andrew Books.

Altman, D. (1982). *The homosexualization of America*. New York: Beacon.

Auerswald, E. H. (1968). Interdisciplinary vs. ecological approach. *Family Process, 7*, 202-215.

Beavers, W. R. (1982). Healthy, midrange, and severely dysfunctional families. In F. Walsh (Ed.), *Normal family processes*. New York: Guilford Press.

Becker, E. (1973). *The denial of death*. New York: Free Press.

Bluebond, L. M. (1978). *The private world of dying children*. New Jersey: Princeton Press.

Boszormenyi-Nagy, I., & Spark, G. (1973). *Invisible loyalties*. New York: Harper & Row.

Bowen, M. (1978). *Family therapy and clinical practice*. New York: Jason Aronson.

Callen, M. (Ed.). (1987). *Surviving and thriving with AIDS*. New York: Michael Hersch Publishers.

Carl, D. (1986). Acquired Immune Deficiency Syndrome: A preliminary examination of the effects on gay couples and coupling. *Journal of Marital and Family Therapy, 12*(3), 241-247.

Carter, E. A., & McGoldrick, M. (Eds.). (1988). *The family life cycle: A framework for family therapy*. 2nd ed. New York: Gardner Press.

Centers for Disease Control. (1987). Human Immunodeficiency Virus infection in the United States: A review of current knowledge. *Morbidity and Mortality Weekly Report, 36*, (Suppl. No. 506), 1-48.

Cleveland, P. H., Walters, L. H., Skeen, P., & Robinson, B. E. (1988). If your child had AIDS . . . : Responses of parents with homosexual children. *Family Relations, 37*, 150-153.

Coleman, E. (1982a). Bisexual and gay men in heterosexual marriage: Conflicts and resolutions in therapy. In J. Gonsiorek (Ed.), *Guide to psychotherapy of gay and lesbian clients*. New York: Haworth Press.

Coleman, E. (1982b). Developmental stages in the coming out process. In J. Gonsiorek (Ed.), *Guide to psychotherapy of gay and lesbian clients*. New York: Haworth Press.

Combrinck-Graham, L. (1985). A developmental model for family systems. *Family Process, 24*(2), 139-150.

Cooper, E. R. (1988, Winter/Spring). AIDS in children: An overview of the medical, epidemiological, and public health problems. *New England Journal of Public Policy, 4*(1), 121-133.

Duvall, E. (1977). *Marriage and family development*. Philadelphia: Lippencott.

Framo, J. (1976). Family of origin as therapeutic resource for adults in marital and family therapy. *Family Process, 15,* 193-210.

Gilbert, J. (1988, January). Coming to terms. *Family Therapy Networker, 12*(1), 42-43, 81.

Goffman, E. (1963). *Stigma: Notes on the management of spoiled identity*. Englewood Cliffs: Prentice-Hall.

Helmquist, M. (1984). *The family guide to AIDS: Responding with your heart*. San Francisco: San Francisco AIDS Foundation.

Herz, F. (1988). The impact of death and serious illness on the family life cycle. In E. A. Carter & M. McGoldrick (Eds.), *The family life cycle*. 2nd ed. New York: Gardner Press.

Hughes, A. M., & O'Neil, M. (1987). Psychosocial assessment and intervention for the person with AIDS. In *AIDS home care and hospice manual*. San Francisco: Visiting Nurses and Hospice of San Francisco.

Imber-Black, E. (1988). *Families and larger systems*. New York: Guilford Press.

Kaplan, L. (1988, January). AIDS and guilt. *Family Therapy Networker, 12*(1), 40-41, 80.

McGoldrick, M., & Gerson, R. (1985). *Genograms in family assessment*. New York: Norton Press.

McGoldrick, M., & Walsh, S. (1983). A systemic view of family history and loss. In M. Aronson & L. Wolberg (Eds.), *Group and family therapy*. New York: Brunner/Mazel.

McGoldrick, M., Pearce, J., & Giordano, J. (Eds.). (1980). *Ethnicity and family therapy*. New York: Guilford Press.

McWhirter, D., & Mattison, A. (1984). *The male couple*. New York: Prentice Hall.

Mohr, R. (1988, January). Deciding what's do-able. *Family Therapy Networker, 12*(1), 34-36.

Moos, R. H. (Ed.). (1984). *Coping with physical illness: Two new perspectives*. New York: Plenum.

Myers, M. (1982). Counseling the parents of young homosexual male patients. In J. Gonsiorek (Ed.), *A guide to psychotherapy with gay and lesbian clients*. New York: Haworth Press.

Neugarten, B. (1976). Adaptation and the life cycle. *Counseling Psychologist, 1,* 16-20.

Patten, J. (1988, January). AIDS and the gay couple. *Family Therapy Networker, 12*(1), 37-39.

Penn, P. (1983). Coalitions and binding interactions in families with chronic illness. *Family Systems Medicine, 1*(1), 16-25.

Rolland J. S. (1984). Toward a psychosocial typology of chronic and life-threatening illness. *Family Systems Medicine, 2*(3), 245-263.

Rolland, J. S. (1987a). Family systems and chronic illness: A typological model. *Journal of Psychotherapy & the Family*, *3*, 143-168.

Rolland, J. S. (1987b). Family illness paradigms: Evolution and significance. *Family Systems Medicine*, *5*(4), 482-503.

Rolland, J. S. (1987c). Chronic illness and the life cycle: A conceptual framework. *Family Process*, *26*(2), 203-221.

Schoen, K. (1986). Psychosocial aspects of hospice care for AIDS patients. *The American Journal of Hospice Care*, *3*, 32-34.

Shanfield, S. B., Benjamin, A. H., & Swaim, B. J. (1984). Parents' reactions to the death of an adult child from cancer. *American Journal of Psychiatry*, *141*, 1092-1094.

Stanton, M. D., Todd, T., & Associates. (1982). *The family therapy of drug abuse and addiction*. New York: Guilford Press.

Tiblier, K. (1987). Intervening with families with young adults with AIDS. In M. Wright & M. L. Leahey (Eds.), *Families and life-threatening illness*. St Louis: Springhouse.

United States Department of Health and Human Services, Public Health Service. (1987). *Report of the Surgeon General's workshop on children with HIV infections and their families*. Washington, DC: U.S. Government Printing Office.

Urwin, C. A. (1988). AIDS in children: A family concern. *Family Relations*, *37*, 154-159.

Walker, G. (1987, April/June). AIDS and family therapy. *Family Therapy Today*, *2*(4,6).

Walker, G. (1988, January). An AIDS journal. *Family Therapy Networker*, *12*(1), 20-33.

Weeks, J. (1985). *Sexuality and its discontents: Meanings and myths and modern sexualities*. London: Rutledge and Kegan Paul.

RESOURCES

AIDS Project
Ackerman Institute for Family Therapy
149 East 78th Street
New York, NY 10021
(212) 879-4900

Gay Men's Health Crisis, Inc.
Box 274
132 West 24th Street
New York, NY 10011
(212) 807-6655/7517

National Hospice Organization
1901 North Moore Street
901
Arlington, VA 22209-1706
(Current listing of hospices
are available.)
(703) 243-5900

Shanti Project
525 Howard Street
San Francisco, CA 94105
(415) 777-2273
(Provides counseling and support
groups for persons with AIDS,
their families, lovers, and friends.)

Visiting Nurses and Hospice of San Francisco
Fox Plaza
1390 Market Street, Suite 510
San Francisco, CA 94102
(415) 861-8705
(Publishes AIDS Home-care
and Hospice Manual).

Women's AIDS Network
San Francisco AIDS Foundation
333 Valencia Street
4th Floor
San Francisco, CA 94103
(415) 863-AIDS

Chapter 4

Societal Implications of AIDS and HIV Infection: HIV Antibody Testing, Health Care, and AIDS Education

D. Bruce Carter, PhD

The AIDS epidemic touches nearly all persons in one way or another (cf. Carter, 1986, 1987). Not only has this disease been prominently featured in the news, in theater, and in movies, but the lives of thousands of persons have been altered by the illness or death of friends, relatives, lovers, and spouses as a result of AIDS and human immunodeficiency virus (HIV) infection. Among those affected by the epidemic are the following: HIV-infected persons and their family members, lovers, and friends; persons who are frightened or confused by media reports on the epidemic; the tax-paying citizen who carries some part of the financial burden associated with studying and treating this disease; and professionals such as doctors, nurses, ministers, social workers, and therapists who are called upon to alleviate the distress associated with the disease.

AIDS and HIV-related diseases have galvanized and polarized families, communities, and agencies throughout the world. AIDS has had a powerful impact on the gay population, creating a new sense of unity and community, affecting significant changes in sexual interactions (Ginzburg, Fleming, & Miller, 1988), and increas-

D. Bruce Carter is Associate Professor of Psychology, Department of Psychology, 430 Huntington Hall, Syracuse University, Syracuse, NY 13244-2340.

129

ing stigmatization and stereotyping (e.g., see Altman, 1986; Nungesser, 1986). Within the political community, debate over alternative approaches to the education of both the general population and, more particularly, children and adolescents about AIDS led to major splits within the Reagan administration. Cabinet level disagreements about the role of the federal government in AIDS education pitted Surgeon General Koop, advocate of secondary school education about AIDS and safer sexual activities (Koop, 1987), against Secretary of Education Bennett, who advocated abstinence and avoidance of drugs as the primary means of reducing HIV infection and AIDS in the general population (Barol, Hager, & Wingert, 1987). Moreover, some gay rights activists and civil libertarians, traditional allies, remain at odds over the acceptability of mandatory testing for antibodies to HIV in selected populations. Although many traditional civil libertarians reject mandatory testing of *any* group as an invasion of privacy, some gay activists support mandatory HIV antibody testing of prison inmates and immigrants to the United States while rejecting mandatory testing of gay men and bisexuals. Clearly the issues surrounding AIDS strike deep at the heart of well-entrenched values at all points along the political continuum and are likely to engender controversy at all levels of society.

This chapter focuses on three major social issues growing out of the AIDS epidemic: HIV antibody testing, medical and psychological care, and education, and on how different sectors of U.S. society have responded to these issues. The section on antibody testing focuses on ways in which individuals, their relationship partners, their families, and their support systems are affected by the results of these tests and concludes with a discussion of the mandatory testing issue for purposes of illustrating the complexity of societal responses to AIDS and HIV infection. The second section on medical and psychological care discusses the health-care needs of persons infected with HIV or at risk for infection and the responses of health-care and mental health professionals. The third section focuses on issues involved in AIDS education, specifically on ways in which the need for explicit and accurate information on HIV transmission conflicts with the traditional views of the American public on sex and sexuality.

HIV ANTIBODY TESTING

Perhaps no issue surrounding AIDS is more controversial than the issue of testing to determine whether or not a person is infected with HIV. This is done by identifying an antibody response to HIV infection (i.e., when presence of antibodies is detected, it is said that the person has seroconverted, become HIV "seropositive," or is "antibody positive"). Public health officials, physicians, politicians, and the public appear polarized by this issue.

In any complex issue, however, there are areas of professional agreement and others in which no definitive answer has emerged. For example, although there is widespread agreement among virtually all professionals that HIV antibody testing can be a useful tool in prevention and treatment, controversy still rages over the way in which such testing should be conducted (anonymously, confidentially, routinely, or in a mandatory fashion) and the ways in which the results of antibody tests should be used. Should a seropositive antibody test result be shared only with the individual testee or is there an obligation to share this information with such persons as medical personnel responsible for care or with sexual partners who may be at risk for infection? Should results be used for sexual contact tracing, as is the case with other sexually transmissible diseases (STDs), or as a basis for denying insurance, housing, or health care? Because the controversy around testing for HIV antibodies encapsulates the major dilemmas that pervade societal responses to AIDS, and because a seropositive response on an HIV antibody test (as with a diagnosis of full-blown or frank AIDS) raises a variety of issues for individuals and their intimate associates, this chapter will focus extensively on antibody testing and its consequences.

The Microscopic Perspective: Implications for Individuals and Families

Antibody tests for HIV and the psychological and social consequences of such testing present an array of issues, both for the individuals who undergo such testing and for their families and loved ones. The decision to undertake an HIV antibody test is often an agonizing one. The possibility of HIV antibody testing often requires that persons admit to themselves that they have engaged in behaviors that have put them at risk for HIV infection, a difficult step for many people because it calls into question their current and future health status. The next step is the decision about where one will go for testing. State and county-funded clinics may offer anonymity, but often are perceived as resources for low-income persons. On the other hand, requesting testing from a private physician may raise anxieties about revealing why the test is sought or how one became infected. Finally, receiving a positive antibody test result will have serious consequences for relationships, behavior patterns, and life plans, and the accompanying despair may undermine commitment to health-promoting behaviors.

Because the decision to be tested and the results of the test affect so dramatically both the individuals who choose to take the test and the lives of those closest to them, and because professionals responsible for assisting persons in these decisions need to be fully informed about the tests, a brief description of the tests and their characteristics appears below.

Description of HIV Antibody Testing

The most commonly used method to detect antibodies to HIV is the Enzyme-Linked Immunosorbent Assay (ELISA). The ELISA is a fairly inexpensive test to administer, costing approximately $3-$10 per test (Howe, 1988; Rothstein, 1987). Because the ELISA was initially developed to screen donated blood, it is an extremely sensitive measure, resulting in accuracy problems. About 50% to 60% of positive responses on an initial ELISA will prove negative on a second ELISA, depending on the seroprevalence rate of the population being tested. If a blood sample is positive on two ELISA tests, confirmatory tests, such as the Western Blot which identifies antibodies to proteins of a specific molecular weight, are generally employed. These tests are more expensive, costing around $65-$100 per test (Howe, 1988) but are effective in eliminating false positives (Rothstein, 1987). Because it takes 6-8 weeks or longer for the body to develop antibodies in sufficient quantities to be detected by these tests, it also is possible to obtain false negative results (i.e., the test result indicates no antibodies even though infection actually has occurred). It is estimated that the false negative rate is 1 in 45,000 or less (Koop, 1987).

It is important to note that the tests currently available do not test for the presence of AIDS or ARC. AIDS and ARC are medical conditions that are diagnosed under specific guidelines originally established by the Centers for Disease Control in 1982 and periodically revised and expanded (e.g., Centers for Disease Control, 1987b). A variety of disease conditions (e.g., Pneumocystis carinii pneumonia, brain lymphomas, and Kaposi's sarcoma) in either the presence or absence of a seropositive test result may be diagnostic of AIDS. Antibody tests may be used as an adjunct diagnostic tool, but are not, of themselves, sufficient to diagnose AIDS or ARC. It is also important to recognize that not all individuals who test seropositive will necessarily go on to develop either AIDS or ARC. Although the estimates for the number of seropositive individuals who will progress to develop AIDS or ARC have been revised steadily upwards (currently ranging between 50% and 90%), some groups of seropositive individuals appear less likely to develop AIDS or ARC than others. For example, although up to 80% of all adult hemophiliacs in the United States are estimated to be HIV seropositive, less than 2% of these individuals have progressed to develop full-blown AIDS (Institute of Medicine, National Academy of Sciences, 1986a).

Because antibody test results are often misunderstood by those receiving them and may have profound emotional consequences, pre- and post-test counseling of testees is recommended (e.g., Dlugosch, Gold, & Dilley, 1986a, 1986b) and is even mandated in certain states. Pre-test counseling usually involves apprising the potential testee, prior to the drawing of blood, of the types of information the test will yield. This counseling insures that the client is able to make a fully informed decision about taking the test and that the person's expectations regarding the test are accurate. This initial counseling session also provides an opportunity for risk-reduction education of the client. Because the test results, whether positive or negative, are likely to have a significant impact on the life and lifestyle of the testee, disclosure of the results of an HIV antibody test should be performed in the context of a counseling session. At this time, clinicians alert the client to possible emotional reactions to the test results, discuss ways to cope with potential relationship disruptions, and help the client begin to plan for necessary behavior changes and medical care. Medical and psychological follow-up, especially for clients who are seropositive, can be planned during this post-test counseling session.

Coping with the Diagnosis

The results of an HIV antibody test have an impact far beyond the individual receiving the test result. Either a positive or a negative test result is likely to have an impact on that individual's relationships with other persons, particularly those with whom the person is sexually or emotionally involved. Seropositive test results certainly will require significant behavioral changes in those who have not modified their sexual behaviors already. Even a seronegative test result may result in behavioral change in non-monogamous couples or sexually active single individuals. In situations in which only one partner in a relationship is HIV infected, psychotherapy for both partners may be required in order to help them cope with issues arising from the revelation of the infection.

Part of the stress involved in receiving a positive antibody test is the awareness that HIV infection often results from behaviors (e.g., sexual intercourse and intravenous drug usage) that are unacceptable to the majority culture. Moreover, such activities may have been conducted outside of the primary relationship, unbeknownst to the uninfected partner. This may be particularly true of bisexual or homosexual men who are heterosexually married but homosexually active. Estimates of the number of these individuals range from 17% to 54% of adult gay males (e.g., Ross, 1983). Moreover, a rising number of cases of HIV infection among heterosexuals has occurred among the partners of male IV drug users (e.g., Green, 1987; Leishman, 1987a). Given the prevalence of HIV infection in both the homosexual and IV drug-using communities, it is likely that gay or drug-using persons may have become infected through behaviors which they were unaware were unsafe and, hence, unintentionally infected their unsuspecting sexual partner.

The diagnosis of HIV infection in a person engaged in a casual sexual relationship (e.g., dating) is likely to have very different effects on both the individuals and the relationship than would be the case if the person were in a committed relationship (e.g., marriage). Among persons who are dating casually, where the level of commitment is low, termination of the relationship often results. In marital relationships and other forms of permanent partnership, both uninfected and infected partners may face a variety of issues and accompanying psychological problems. For example, in the case of the married bisexual or homosexual male, the wife may be unaware of her husband's extramarital sexual activities or of his sexual orientation. Therefore, she must deal simultaneously with his sexual orientation, his nonfidelity, and his HIV infection. Moreover, the sexual partners of HIV-infected individuals often must consider significant changes in joint sexual activities regardless of their current state of infection, given that repeated exposure to the virus may influence the progression of the disease (e.g., Institute of Medicine, National Academy of Sciences, 1986a, 1986b).

Discovery of the infection of a presumably monogamous spouse is likely to raise significant issues for relationships. Fear, guilt, and anger are likely to become paramount (e.g., Interrante, 1987; Martelli, Peltz, & Messina, 1987; Moffatt, 1986) even in relationships in which the mode of HIV transmission was neither sexual nor through IV needle sharing. For example, in order to prevent potential infection of the uninfected partner, they may avoid all forms of physical expression of love for one another. There may be bitterness and guilt if the partner at identifiable risk (e.g., the gay or IV drug-using spouse) infects the other partner (e.g., the wife who is unaware of her husband's extramarital relationships or activities). As a consequence, couples in committed relationships may need therapeutic assistance in order to cope with the relationship issues resulting from or stimulated by the HIV infection.

The diagnosis of HIV seropositivity, with its potential for subsequent AIDS, has effects extending beyond the immediate couple relationship to relationships with members of the individuals' families and friends. For example, persons who have AIDS or are HIV infected frequently find that their support systems and friendship networks dissolve as a consequence of their diagnosis (e.g., Nichols, 1986), resulting in feelings of isolation and loneliness, depression, and rejection. Relationships with family members often become progressively strained (e.g., Moffatt, 1986; Peabody, 1986), a tendency that is likely to be exacerbated if the basis for the infection was previously unknown to or hidden from the family (e.g., Shilts, 1987). Moreover, even in families where issues such as the sexual orientation of a family member have been dealt with, diagnosis of HIV infection or AIDS is likely to lead to a reemergence of tensions and problems (see Shilts, 1987 for examples). As a consequence, a diagnosis of HIV seropositivity is likely to result in disruption of the family unit, either the biological/legal unit most frequently defined as family and/or the close and binding relationships self-defined as family. Thus, at the very time when stress may be highest for the family and its members, and when there is the greatest need for access to the unified resources of the family, the family may, in fact, be torn apart by the conflicts resulting from the diagnosis.

The negative consequences of seropositivity are likely to be greatest in community settings where fears of exposure by infected persons are greatest. For example, there may be unreasoning fears that gay or bisexual waiters and cooks may transmit the virus in the course of their foodhandling or that co-workers, known or suspected to be gay, may be infected and thus transmit the virus through a variety of unlikely modes such as papercuts. Most telling, perhaps, are the responses of parents to the knowledge or suspicion that HIV-infected children are attending schools with their own children. For example, in Florida a family that included three HIV-infected hemophiliac boys suffered the loss of their home due to a suspicious fire that erupted following a controversy over the boys' attendance at the local public school (e.g., Herald American News Service, 1987; Krauthammer, 1987). The fears of the members of the community that these infected boys might transmit the virus to uninfected children in the school setting far outweighed professionals' abilities to reassure parents that such vectors of transmission were highly unlikely. Indeed, parents and officials expressed little remorse in interviews over the loss of the home or the subsequent exit of the affected family from this semi-rural community (e.g., Herald American News Service, 1987). This is not an isolated incident. Families in other communities have faced varying levels of support or rejection as a result of having an HIV-infected member (see Moffatt, 1986; Peabody, 1986; SerVaas, 1987).

Hysteria and discrimination in response to the presence of persons with AIDS or HIV infection is clearly a factor that affects the degree of support available to persons with AIDS and their families and the chances of preventing further spread of HIV infection (e.g., Institute of Medicine, National Academy of Sciences 1986a, 1986b). Indeed, community support for HIV-infected individuals and their families may be an important determinant of the degree to which persons with AIDS are able to cope with the vicissitudes of the disease itself. AIDS education efforts must be directed at informing the entire community about the modes of HIV transmission and the psychological and emotional costs of the disease for the infected and their loved ones. The information provided in these educational efforts should be accurate, current, sensitive to the concerns of those directly affected by the epidemic, and nonsensational in style. An example of inappropriate media coverage is discussed briefly below.

In 1986, reports surfaced that HIV had been found in the bodies of certain insects (e.g., mosquitos, body lice, and fleas) in Central Africa (e.g., Leishman, 1987b). The ability of scientists to identify virons in these insects led to the hypothesis that an insect transmission vector of HIV would be possible. This hypothesis, in turn, was picked up by the news media and resulted in the reporting that AIDS (not HIV infection!) could be transmitted through an insect vector. Clearly, the scientists involved in the original report were not remiss in reporting their findings nor have the scientists who studied this mode of transmission been unprofessional in pursuing this line of research. Theoretical speculation is clearly part of the scientific method and this particular speculation must be understood in the context of an hypothesis that was advanced and was later proven to be false (e.g., Castro et al., 1988; Koop, 1987). However, this scientific speculation was quickly sensationalized, leading to a widespread fear that insect transmission of HIV was an immediate public health concern (see Leishman, 1987b for one of the least sensationalistic of these reports). Needlessly intensifying the fears of the noninfected population with alerts to fairly unlikely modes of viral transmission (e.g., Crenshaw, 1987; Masters, Johnson, & Kolodny, 1988; Noebel et al., 1987) is unscientific, potentially irresponsible, and may result in intensifying discrimination against HIV-infected individuals and their family members. Unfortunately, sensationalism has been the rule, rather than the exception, in much of the media coverage of the AIDS epidemic.

The Macroscopic Perspective: Responses of Society

Responses to HIV infection at the more macroscopic level of societal institutions reveal the stresses seen at the microscopic levels. Governmental responses to HIV infection among its citizens have included requirements for AIDS education in schools (e.g., "Will Regents'," 1987) and proposals for legislative protection of HIV-infected individuals from discrimination (e.g., Dunne & Lombardi, 1987), as well as calls for mandatory testing and the quarantining of HIV-infected individuals (e.g., Dannemeyer, 1987), an issue covered in greater detail below. Organized religion is an excellent example of the variety of responses to HIV infection and AIDS within mainstream society, and it is to these responses that we now turn our attention.

The Judeo-Christian heritage shared by the majority of U.S. citizens is clear in the messages it presents to members of its synagogues and churches. First, believers are instructed that they are to care for the sick and needy in society, activities that are seen as "good works" by the organized religions. Second, biblical and nonbiblical injunctions state that we should "love the sinner and hate the sin," expressing a need for compassion among believers. These precepts and injunctions, however, break down in the face of HIV infection, in large part because of the behaviors (e.g., anal intercourse, multiple sexual partners, or IV drug use) and the groups associated with the original infection (e.g., drug users and gay men). Issues regarding sexual orientation have been of concern to members of both the Christian and Jewish faiths, and the treatment of gay believers and nonbelievers has been fraught with controversy historically (e.g., Boswell, 1980; McNeil, 1988; Scroggs,

1983). Although the responses of individual congregations to an HIV-infected individual may vary dramatically, the responses of religious hierarchies may be divided into two categories. The responses of fundamentalist and orthodox religions have been fairly negative whereas more mainstream religious groups have tended to call for support for HIV-infected individuals and persons with AIDS. In both instances, dealing with HIV infection has been tainted by the attitudes which these divergent religious groups characteristically have had toward sexuality in general and homosexuality in particular.

It is clear that religion and religious organizations can, do, and will play a major role in societal responses to AIDS. Depending on the denomination and congregation, diagnoses of HIV infection or AIDS may lead to one or more of many possible responses (e.g., Fortunato, 1987). For some, seropositivity is indicative of God's wrath being visited on sinners, as is exemplified frequently in Old Testament writings. Those infected and those who care for infected persons may face either a crisis of faith, questioning the justness of a god who would visit such a pestilence on humanity or themselves, or a renewal of faith, finding the strength through religious belief to bear the psychological turmoil accompanying AIDS. Religious workers called upon to minister to the sick and dying may find themselves confronting individuals whose illness and humanity make them difficult to ignore or dismiss. The AIDS epidemic may result in many religious organizations reexamining their traditional views of homosexuality or may propel them further into intransigence regarding sexuality-related issues.

Because antibody testing and the results of tests have such an enormous impact on individuals, their families, and their communities, it is relevant to examine the issues surrounding mandatory testing as an example of the societal response to HIV infection.

Mandatory versus Voluntary Testing

The questions surrounding mandatory and routine testing for HIV antibodies reflect significant conflicts between the tradition of respect for human rights and civil liberties and public health concerns for protection of noninfected persons. Nowhere was this conflict more obvious than in the responses of persons attending the Third (1987) International Conference on Acquired Immunodeficiency Syndrome to announcements by several federal officials, including then Vice President George Bush, that routine HIV antibody testing would begin soon for inmates in federal prisons, immigrants to the United States, and persons participating in drug detoxification programs. Such announcements were greeted by boos and shouts of disapproval, not only from AIDS activists and gays, but also from members of the scientific research community (cf. Shilts, 1987).

Such disapproval is not indicative of a lack of support for HIV antibody screening per se but rather is a stance against testing of individuals that occurs in either a routine or mandatory fashion. Scientists and health professionals stand united in their belief that all donated blood, semen, and body organs *must* be routinely *screened* for HIV antibodies in order to prevent the spread of infection to persons receiving these lifesaving donations. The controversy over routine and mandatory testing does not focus on screening of these donations but rather focuses on the *testing of individuals.*

Routine testing refers to situations in which all persons are tested for antibodies to HIV either as part of a standard operating procedure or as part of a standardized assessment or treatment protocol. Thus, routine HIV antibody screening can (and does in some states) occur when persons seek treatment at sexually transmissible disease (STD) clinics, drug detoxification programs, and hospitals. Because the tests are administered as part of a larger battery of tests, voluntary, informed consent often is not required and the results of the tests become a part of the person's overall medical record. This allows others, such as insurance companies or governmental agencies, access to information that can be used as the basis for differential treatment (such as health insurance cancellation or denial of medical services). Moreover, routine testing of *all* persons is not the norm. Generally, "routine" testing is done only when the individual is perceived to belong to a "high-risk group" (such as gay men) and thus it is not, by definition, routine but rather discriminatory.

Mandatory testing refers to testing situations in which persons are *required* to be tested in order to receive services or because they fall (or are perceived to fall) into "high-risk groups," such as gay men,

IV drug users, or, less commonly, sexually active persons regardless of their sexual orientations. The fine line distinguishing routine from mandatory testing is defined by the ways in which the test is administered and test results are employed, a line that is frequently crossed. If the testing protocol is standard for all individuals, if compliance is nonvoluntary, if testing occurs over the objections of the individual, or if a test or seronegative result is a prerequisite for receipt of services, then the testing is no longer routine. This fine line between routine and mandatory testing has been crossed by a number of testing programs.

Arguments for Routine or Mandatory Testing

Two arguments have been made in favor of routine and mandatory testing programs. First, it has been argued that such programs would provide more accurate epidemiological data on the size of the AIDS epidemic than is available currently. These data would allow better planning for future AIDS-related health-care needs as well as provide more accurate data on the number of seropositive individuals whose disease progresses to full-blown AIDS. Proposals focusing on epidemiology are perhaps the most reasonable of all those advanced for routine or mandatory screening for two principal reasons. First, in general, epidemiological studies need not obtain information on participants' identities because prevalence of infection is the primary concern. Thus, issues of confidentiality and discrimination become moot, given that adequate precautions are taken to insure the anonymity of participants. Second, for reasons discussed below, research data collected to date on the prevalence of HIV infection in the U.S. population may be biased and there is no way of correcting this without additional epidemiological data.

Currently available estimates for HIV-infection prevalence in the U.S. population are, in fact, merely estimates (e.g., Adkins, 1986; Associated Press, 1987). Data underlying these estimates are based largely on extrapolations from HIV-infectivity rates found among armed forces enlistees, donors to blood banks, and persons seeking treatment or participating in research at certain hospitals, drug detoxification programs, and STD clinics. Any of these sources could be biased. For example, persons who suspect they are seropositive have been asked not to donate blood and thus may be self-selected out of the population sample drawn from blood banks, resulting in underestimations of HIV-infection prevalence. In contrast, STD clinics may provide an overestimation of seropositivity prevalence because persons attending such clinics probably are sexually active and suspect that they have been exposed to one or more sexually transmissible diseases. Well-formulated studies of HIV-infection prevalence, employing scientifically derived sampling procedures and careful screening, would provide invaluable information on the progression of this epidemic.

One such a study is currently underway in the state of New York. In August of 1987, Governor Mario M. Cuomo announced that New York will be undertaking a $3 million study of HIV-infection prevalence (Cuomo, 1987). The data base will be 100,000 blood samples, not individuals, drawn from persons whose blood is being taken for other diagnostic purposes. Three primary groups of individuals will provide the samples. The first group will be persons enrolled in drug detoxification programs. Rates of seropositivity in this group will provide estimates of the numbers of IV drug users who are currently HIV infected. The second group will be persons attending county STD clinics in the state. Data from this group will provide information on rates of seropositivity among sexually active individuals. Finally, the third group will be newborn infants. At birth, newborn infants' antibodies generally duplicate those of their mothers. Thus, data from this group will give an indication of the number of women infected with HIV. In all instances, full confidentiality and anonymity is guaranteed for those providing blood samples. It is Cuomo's hope that the resulting data will allow the state of New York, home to the single largest group of AIDS patients, to make "sound public health policy decisions" (Cuomo, 1987, p. 11).

Although Cuomo's plan for this epidemiological study is commendable, several problems remain. First, it is unclear whether persons from whom blood is drawn will be voluntary participants who are aware they are participating in this study or are persons who simply will provide blood for other purposes, unaware that they are part of this epidemiological study. Clearly, certain ethical issues arise if standards of informed consent are violated in this study but to require informed consent might result in a biased sample. Second, it remains unclear from both the Governor's statements and from subsequent press reports whether seropositive persons will be informed of their antibody status. Clearly, such information would be valuable for such individuals to have, but provision of such information may be impossible given the desire to insure anonymity and persons would have to make an informed decision about receiving their test results. Despite these minor flaws and ethical concerns, this undertaking by the state of New York may provide us with the best information possible on the prevalence of HIV infection in the general population.

A second major argument for mandatory testing is that it would serve to control further spread of HIV infection among the noninfected population. For example, in 1987, Congressional Representative William Dannemeyer (R-California) introduced a series of bills that would have required mandatory testing of inmates in federal prisons, immigrants to the United States, persons arrested for prostitution or drug-related crimes, and all persons seeking to be married. Although Rep. Dannemeyer noted that the first line of defense in dealing with antibody positive individuals should be counseling, he proposed that legal restrictions, including "court sanctioned isolation," be imposed on those who failed to modify their behavior to reduce HIV transmission (Dannemeyer, 1987).

Dangers of Mandatory and Routine Testing

What is potentially insidious about mandatory testing is not the testing itself, but the consequences resulting from such testing. The twin dangers of routine testing are (a) it would become mandatory for particular groups of people and (b) the results of the tests would be used as a basis for discriminating against those persons who test seropositive. For example, military recruits who test positive are discharged as are seropositive active duty personnel who admit engaging in homosexuality or IV drug use. Hospitals could refuse treatment of routinely screened antibody positive individuals and have, in fact, done so (e.g., Harris, 1987). Secretary of Education Bennett suggested that HIV positive prisoners awaiting parole or discharge remain incarcerated as a result of their antibody status.

Finally, in states (e.g., Illinois and Louisiana, "Broad AIDS laws," 1987) where routine testing is conducted on marriage license applicants, a seropositive result on the test of one or both partners may preclude the couple from receiving a marriage license.

Complex social issues arise out of mandatory testing programs. For example, it remains unclear what states would do to insure that couples refused a marriage license on the basis of a seropositive test result would not engage in unprotected sexual contact in the absence of a marriage license or certificate. Are we to reinstitute long-abandoned (or long-ignored) laws prohibiting cohabitation in the absence of marriage? How will we deal with couples in which only one person is infected? Will we encourage them to dissolve their relationship or, instead, help them adjust to the changes inherent in any intensive relationship with a person with HIV infection/AIDS? In a similar vein, routine screening of hospital patients, especially surgical patients, has been suggested, a recommendation that raises a variety of issues relevant to access to medical care. For example, although it is apparent that physicians could refuse to perform elective medical procedures on HIV-infected patients, the ethical issues surrounding a physician's refusal to perform nonelective procedures (such as life-saving surgery) are myriad (e.g., "AIDS suspicion bars surgery," 1987).

A number of persons have advocated using the results of antibody tests and/or membership in high-risk groups as a means of creating an "AIDS-free zone" in the United States. In order to control what are perceived as the twin roots of the AIDS problem, homosexuality and drug abuse, Paul Cameron (e.g., Noebel, Cameron, & Lutton, 1987) has advocated imposing penalties on any state, municipality, or institution of higher learning that recognizes the civil rights of gays, provides office space or facilities for any pro-homosexual group, or permits an openly homosexual individual to receive payment for services of any kind. Cameron further advocates that homosexuality and drug abuse be made violations of state and federal laws. Although Rep. Dannemeyer's call for mandatory testing and Cameron's call for eliminating AIDS through elimination of homosexuality and drug abuse differ on the issue of counseling individuals at risk or who test positive on the antibody test, incarceration would be one outcome of either proposal.

At first glance, Cameron's (e.g., Noebel et al., 1987) proposals may appear more unreasonable than those proposed by Dannemeyer. However, a careful consideration of the implications of both sets of proposals uncovers the major issue underlying all forms of routine or mandatory testing. Specifically, over the long run, what is to be done with the millions of individuals who test antibody positive or who are homosexual men or substance abusers?

Several solutions to this problem have been proposed with great sincerity. For example, in Congressional testimony, Dr. William O'Connor, a California physician, suggested that all HIV-positive individuals be quarantined on the Hawaiian island of Molokai, a former leper colony (Walter, 1987). Similarly, Dr. Vernon Mark, a neurosurgeon of the Harvard Medical School, has suggested that "carriers of AIDS who persist in spreading it" should be quarantined on an island in Massachusetts Bay that also was formerly a leper colony (Foreman, 1986, p. 30). For weeks after Dr. Mark's comments appeared in print, gay men in New York City sang "I'll take Manhattan" in mocking recognition of these and similar comments on quarantining by other individuals. Other persons, such as columnist William F. Buckley, have suggested that seropositive individuals be marked in a permanent fashion, such as a tattoo on the buttocks for seropositive gay men, warning noninfected persons that they were dealing with an infected individual. Although Buckley's suggestion of tattooing seropositive individuals, which he compared to the yellow Stars of David employed by Nazis in concentration camps to identify Jewish inmates, was later retracted, the fact that such statements appeared in a nationally syndicated column is, itself, disturbing.

Although some may scoff at such suggestions as the rantings of the bigoted or the uninformed, the prospect for quarantine for some portion of the infected or at-risk population remains distressingly high. For example, Mayo (1988) has stated that it is conceivable that courts may be able to order the indefinite incarceration or quarantining of "recalcitrant" antibody-positive individuals simply by relying on the public health laws existing in many states. He notes, however, that such attempts would face both constitutional and ethical scrutiny. In this vein, a New York City judge hearing a case on whether a child with AIDS would be allowed to attend a public school noted that he could not imagine why the city health department did not quarantine adults with advanced AIDS.

In some states, attempts to legislate quarantine measures for persons with AIDS and/or seropositive individuals have received dramatic public support. For example, in California in 1986 the La-Rouche AIDS Initiative, which would have mandated antibody testing for persons at risk and the quarantining of all seropositive individuals, was placed on the election ballot with well over 700,000 signatures (Kreiger & Appleman, 1986). It has been estimated that the LaRouche proposal would have cost over $2.3 billion in economic output and an additional $630 million in tax revenues, while depriving, conservatively, over 300,000 Californians of their civil rights (McGrath & Sutcliffe, 1986). Although this referendum proposal was later defeated by a 62% to 38% vote margin, the mere fact that so many people supported and voted for this proposal is alarming.

The question that remains unaddressed by those supporting quarantine measures is what happens to those who are quarantined. How will we, as a society, provide for the health care of desperately ill persons whom we have incarcerated to protect ourselves from them? Will we rely on religious workers and other volunteers who, like the valiant men and women who cared for the lepers of past generations, give up their lives in the uninfected world to live with these whom society has expelled? Or will we simply allow such persons to live and die in colonies without providing for their care? How will we decide which persons are to be forced to participate in mandatory testing programs? Will we, as some insurance companies have already done, consider that all unmarried men over the age of 25 living in "high-risk zones" (e.g., San Francisco, New York City, Greenwich Village) or engaged in suspicious occupations (e.g., hairdressers, dancers), or all persons who fail to match conventional norms for masculine behavior, are under suspicion of being gay and, hence, at risk for infection? And where will we put the estimated 271,000 cases of AIDS and the 10 million individuals who the Centers for Disease Control have predicted will become infected by 1991? None of these questions are addressed by those advocating quarantine. They seem content simply to shut infected persons away from the noninfected community.

The clearest danger of mandatory or routine HIV antibody testing is a gradual march from testing to isolation to quarantine. A two-tiered society would be created of infected and at-risk-for-infection persons versus the uninfected individuals, that is, the noninfected "us" versus the infected "them." Clearly, such a dichotomy would not bode well for society at large (Hammonds, 1987). Moreover, as the psychological distance between "us" and "them" became more dramatic, even more draconian measures than those suggested above would become possible.

Other fairly convincing arguments have been marshaled against the use of mandatory testing for HIV. For example, a number of scientists (e.g., Health and Public Policy Committee of the American College of Physicians & the Infectious Diseases Society of America, 1986; Institute of Medicine, National Academy of Sciences, 1986a, 1986b) have expressed concern that implementing routine or mandatory antibody testing would result in persons at risk for infection "going underground," thus facilitating the further spread of the epidemic. Moreover, it is clearly the case that our resources for providing counseling for the large number of persons who potentially would be tested are inadequate. Thus, the educational interventions for infected persons and the provision of assistance in coping with positive or negative test results that could be provided by post-test counseling would be lost. Finally, as the number of persons being tested increases, the potential for false positive results on HIV antibody tests also increases. Thus, mandatory testing of members of high-risk groups or the population at large might overwhelm an already overburdened system.

The strongest argument against either routine or mandatory testing comes from physicians, medical researchers, public health administrators, and the Surgeon General of the United States. As with a single voice, these individuals have stated that routine or mandatory testing is not advisable because *it is not medically indicated* (cf. Centers for Disease Control, 1987a; Health and Public Policy Committee of the American College of Physicians & the Infectious Diseases Society of America, 1986; Institute of Medicine, National Academy of Sciences, 1986a; Koop, 1987). According to these experts, because persons may be HIV-infected yet remain HIV-seronegative and because a wide range of serious illnesses other than

HIV infection may be blood borne, all persons should be treated as though they can transmit disease through their blood or other body fluids. Thus, in health-care settings, universal blood/body fluids precautions (such as the use of masks, gowns, and latex gloves) are advised for those dealing with potentially infectious body fluids of any and all patients (Health and Public Policy Committee of the American College of Physicians & the Infectious Diseases Society of America, 1986; Institute of Medicine, National Academy of Sciences, 1986a; Koop, 1987). Universal use of blood/body fluid precautions should substantially reduce the possibility of transmission of HIV and other infectious agents in settings where blood-to-blood transmission is most likely to occur, the major argument advanced for routine testing. Moreover, in the absence of an effective drug, treatment, or vaccine, little can be done medically to ameliorate the symptoms of those persons identified as being infected with HIV. Thus it is feared that the primary use of either routine or mandatory testing of individuals will result in discrimination against seropositive individuals rather than in the provision of treatment (e.g., Health and Public Policy Committee of the American College of Physicians & the Infectious Diseases Society of America, 1986; Institute of Medicine, National Academy of Sciences, 1986a, 1986b).

Conclusion

Review of the issues surrounding antibody testing makes it clear that, as proposed by the vast majority of public health experts and AIDS researchers (e.g., Koop, 1987; Krim, 1987), there is a definite need for *routine screening of blood, semen and donated organs* and for *voluntary and confidential testing of individuals* for antibodies to HIV. Such testing should be readily available at minimal or no cost, and information about testing programs and procedures should be distributed widely so that persons whose behavior has put them at risk for HIV infection can determine their antibody status. It is equally apparent that, because of the potential economic and social costs and because there is no available vaccine or cure for AIDS or HIV infection, *routine or mandatory testing of individuals is unwarranted for any reason*. It also is clear that both pre- and post-test counseling should be important components of any antibody testing program. This will require that medical professionals (e.g., physicians, nurses, and dentists) receive additional training to facilitate their comfort in dealing with issues surrounding HIV antibody testing. Finally, legislation protecting the rights of seropositive individuals is needed because such persons may suffer discrimination as a result of their antibody status (Christensen & Ringel, 1986; d'Adesky, 1987; Dunne & Lombardi, 1987; Lambda Legal Defense Fund, 1987). Although there undoubtedly will be, from time to time, a few seropositive individuals who engage in behaviors that put other persons at risk for HIV infection, regulations to allow public health officials to monitor and perhaps restrict the behavior of such persons already exist in the public health codes of most states. Thus, no further legislation seems necessary to facilitate such surveillance (Macklin, 1986).

HEALTH CARE ISSUES

Imperative in any discussion of the impact of AIDS on society is a discussion of the impact of the disease on the health-care community. Questions arise regarding medical and mental health care for persons who are HIV-infected or have AIDS, supports for relationship partners and family members, and the economic costs of addressing these physical and psychological health-related issues. In addition, AIDS raises important ethical and moral issues for health-care professionals.

The responses of the medical and mental health communities to AIDS have been, on the whole, mixed. Although the medical and psychological needs of persons with AIDS are in some ways similar to those of other patients with catastrophic or terminal illnesses, AIDS and HIV infection present problems that are distinct from those seen in other illnesses (e.g., Institute of Medicine, National Academy of Sciences, 1986a, 1986b; Kübler-Ross, 1987). Persons concerned with the physical health of persons with AIDS (e.g., doctors, nurses, dentists, and laboratory technicians) may find themselves confronting psychological issues for which their training has ill-prepared them. Similarly, mental health professionals (psychologists, family therapists, social workers, and counselors) may find themselves at a loss to deal with the physiological problems, such as neurological dysfunctions, resulting from HIV infection. The major societal issues related to health care are discussed in three sections: physical health care, mental health care, and the costs of health care.

Physical Health Care

Of particular concern to HIV-infected persons and their families is the issue of access to adequate medical care and humane delivery of services. Persons with AIDS worry that they will be denied medical care or will not receive sufficient care due to professionals' fears about the disease or attitudes regarding persons in the identified "risk groups." Fears about denial of health care are not unwarranted. In a number of metropolitan areas, persons with AIDS have been denied treatment by health-care professionals, both directly and indirectly. For example, some ambulance companies and volunteer fire departments have kept lists of persons with, or suspected to have, AIDS and have instructed drivers not to answer or "to drive slowly" in response to calls from particular addresses. Humane delivery of health care is also an issue. The fact that health-care workers may wear masks, gowns, and latex gloves when dealing with an HIV-infected person sometimes is experienced as dehumanizing by the patient. This section will focus on the following issues that affect access to adequate and humane physical care: availability of drug treatments for HIV infection, vaccines against the HIV infection, and the risks for and attitudes of caregivers that affect treatment.

Drug Treatments

Although clinical trials of a number of drugs are ongoing, currently only one drug is licensed by the U.S. Food and Drug Administration (FDA) for treatment of HIV infection: Azidothymidine (AZT or Retrovir). AZT interferes with the replication of HIV, slowing or halting the growth of the virus in persons with AIDS and AIDS-related conditions (ARC). The efficacy of this drug has been demonstrated by decreases in the rate of opportunistic infections and an increase in the longevity of persons receiving AZT relative to those not receiving the drug (e.g., Fischl et al., 1987). Unfortunately, to date, little data exist on the efficacy of AZT in the treatment of persons who are HIV seropositive but otherwise asymptomatic. In general, drugs such as AZT, show high levels of toxicity (i.e., have debilitating effects on the functioning of major organ systems), and it may or may not be advisable for asymptomatic HIV-seropositive persons to take such medications (e.g., Osborn, 1987). In the absence of definitive research, it is difficult to say whether the use of antiviral drugs, such as AZT, in the treatment of asymptomatic seropositive individuals would be effective.

AZT is an expensive drug to take, averaging $10,000 per year per patient (Micheli, 1987). For the most part, persons taking this drug are persons with AIDS who are disabled as a result of their condition and, thus, are covered by federal or state medical programs such as Medicaid or New York State's AIDS Drug Assistance Program (ADAP). As a result, the direct cost of medication is, most often, borne by neither the patient nor by private insurance. However, it is clear that the cost of AZT for all persons currently diagnosed as having AIDS would be extraordinary. If all of the approximately 20,000 living cases of AIDS were taking AZT, the cost would be $200 million per year for AZT alone. This cost would not include other medical costs arising over the course of the disease (e.g., hospital care for treatment of the side effects of AZT and for opportunistic infections), estimated to be $94,000 per patient (Harris, 1987; Micheli, 1987). Thus, the cost of AZT, even if only used for persons with AIDS, is potentially prohibitive. The cost of implementing programs providing AZT for the estimated 1.5 million or more currently HIV-infected persons in the United States would be in the billions of dollars. Clearly, both governmental and private insurers may be hesitant about paying for a drug treatment that would cost billions and might be of limited effectiveness in halting or postponing development of actual disease.

In reality, it is unclear whether HIV-infected persons who do not have AIDS or ARC would qualify for either private or public assistance to receive AZT when it is taken to prevent or forestall the progression of HIV infection. Although all insurance carriers offer some coverage for medicines used in the treatment of actual disease, many will not cover preventive treatments, such as might be the case in the use of AZT for asymptomatic seropositive persons. Moreover, because HIV infection may never result in actual disease (e.g., "AIDS virus: Always fatal?," 1987), insurance carriers may be unwilling to "bet" the $10,000 per year it would cost to provide each HIV-infected person with AZT. It is clear, also, that most HIV-infected persons would find it difficult to pay the yearly cost of a drug that may or may not prevent the progression of the disease to frank AIDS. Thus, at present, there is no drug that is both affordable and available to asymptomatic seropositive individuals.

AIDS/HIV Vaccines

Although a number of researchers around the world are searching for an HIV vaccine, the prospects for discovering a vaccine remain dim (e.g., Osborn, 1987). A variety of characteristics of HIV, such as its ability to evade the immune system and its high level of genetic mutation (e.g., see chapter on the HIV Epidemic in this volume), would make it difficult to produce a vaccine that would be medically effective against this virus. Additional problems arise when one considers the problems associated with reconstituting the immune systems of persons who have been infected with HIV as a result of the testing of an ineffective vaccine (e.g., Osborn, 1987).

The difficulties that accompany testing and licensing of an HIV vaccine are formidable. First, for a long time HIV appeared to affect human beings almost exclusively. Thus, the use of animal models typical in the development of other medications and vaccines has been difficult (e.g., see chapter on the HIV Epidemic in this volume). As a result, testing of vaccine on humans has appeared to be the only way to determine the effectiveness of such interventions. Second, any potential vaccine would have to be tested on groups of volunteers who would then be tracked to determine whether or not (a) antibody negative individuals seroconverted in response to the vaccine, as would be expected; and (b) vaccinated individuals, or at least a significant proportion of such individuals, did not develop HIV infection as a result of subsequent exposure to the virus.

The ethical problems associated with the use of humans to test a vaccine are obvious. Although exposure of vaccinated individuals to infection is the only means of testing the effectiveness of a vaccine, encouraging or condoning behaviors that would place such individuals at risk for infection in order to ascertain vaccine effectiveness raises at least one clear ethical issue. Without empirical evidence of vaccine effectiveness, governmental approval would be withheld. However, to document such effectiveness would require that volunteer participants engage in behaviors that put them at significant risk for infection if the vaccine is not effective. Although such difficult moral issues should not preclude further research and development of an HIV vaccine, it is clear that researchers must be prepared to address complex ethical issues when determining how they will test the effectiveness of any vaccine developed.

Further complications would arise in the distribution of any potential vaccine. First, persons who might benefit from vaccination would have to be identified and then convinced that vaccination would be of benefit to them. Clearly, given the level of concern exhibited by persons in some "high-risk groups," such as gay men, about the possibility of infection, voluntary participation in such a program might be the simplest of issues to resolve. Other risk groups (e.g., intravenous drug users and married bisexuals) may be more difficult to include in any vaccination program without the imposition of widespread, mandatory vaccination programs — programs that raise other legal and ethical issues. What, for example, is to be done with the gay or bisexual Christian Scientists or Seventh Day Adventists whose religious beliefs may preclude them from submitting to a vaccine but whose behavior may lead to their own and others' subsequent infection?

Perhaps more pertinent are the potential costs associated with complications of immunization in a widespread inoculation program. Instructional here is the example of the federal campaign for immunization against swine-flu implemented in 1976-1977 in the United States. Although the campaign may have been effective, given that the much-touted epidemic never emerged, the cost of claims associated with debilitating reactions to vaccination cost the U.S. government over $4 billion (Osborn, 1987). Comparable costs might be associated with side effects of HIV vaccination programs. Such costs would be over and above the actual cost of researching, developing, and producing a vaccine. Again, although such considerations should not preclude the development and implementation of a vaccine that might save millions of human lives, such concerns must be addressed by both scientists and the public.

At present, the expert opinion is that *education is the best vaccine we have to counter AIDS and HIV infection* (e.g., Carter, 1986; Gostin & Curran, 1986; Green, 1987; Health and Public Policy Committee of the American College of Physicians & the Infectious Diseases Society of America, 1986; Koop, 1987; Waxman, 1987). As discussed extensively elsewhere (e.g., see chapter on Strategies for Education and Prevention in this volume), educational programs that promote behavioral change have been successful in convincing populations at risk to engage in "safer sex" or sexual behaviors that minimize the possibility of viral transmission (e.g., Carter, 1986; Kelly & St. Lawrence, 1986; Martin, 1987).

Risks for Medical Personnel

Health-care practitioners are often deeply concerned with the risk at which they put themselves, and potentially their families, in their delivery of health care. For example, nurses, physicians, and oral surgeons may put themselves at risk for HIV infection by administering procedures (such as surgical procedures) that can lead to a direct infusion of infected blood into their systems. Although perhaps in contradiction to the traditional codes of ethics governing health-care professionals (e.g., the Hippocratic oath of physicians), such concerns are understandable human reactions to a disease that, thus far, has been inevitably fatal. The frustrations that AIDS patients feel when their heretofore all-knowing physician offers them no cure (e.g., Kübler-Ross, 1987) are mirrored in the frustrations of health-care professionals' recognition that their medical skills are inadequate against a disease that can kill them as well.

Although the concerns of health-care professionals about the possibility of HIV transmission are legitimate, it is clearly the case that there is an *ethical obligation on their part not to discriminate in the provision of health care against persons with AIDS or HIV infection or those perceived to be at risk* (Institute of Medicine, National Academy of Sciences, 1986a, 1986b; New York Times News Service, 1987). As noted by the Health and Public Policy Committee of the American College of Physicians & the Infectious Diseases Society of America (1986),

> Health care workers who have the primary responsibility for a patient's well-being must provide high-quality, nonjudgmental care to their patients, even at the risk of contracting a patient's disease. Physicians and nurses are charged by the ethics of their healing professions to treat all patients with all forms of sickness and disease. . . . It is inappropriate for any health care employee to compromise the treatment of patients with transmissible, lethal diseases such as AIDS on the grounds that such patients present unacceptable medical risks. (p. 576)

The obligation to treat AIDS patients and those who are HIV seropositive extends not only to the health-care professionals themselves but to the institutions (i.e., hospitals and clinics) in which medical care is generally provided.

Concerns about HIV transmission in administering routine, noninvasive health care appear to be largely unwarranted. Studies of HIV transmission and seroconversion among family members and other persons whose contact with persons with AIDS was casual (i.e., nonsexual, non-needle-sharing) indicate no seroconversion of persons who had casual contact with infected persons (e.g., Friedland et al., 1986). Moreover, health-care workers who have received needlesticks from hypodermics used in treatment of HIV-infected persons and AIDS patients only rarely have seroconverted and none, to date, has developed AIDS. Indeed, epidemiological studies of HIV infection among health-care workers not at risk for infection due to sexual behaviors or IV-needle sharing indicate that the risk of HIV infection in hospital and clinic settings is extremely small, particularly if stringent infection control measures are taken (e.g., Centers for Disease Control, 1988; Institute of Medicine, National Academy of Sciences, 1986a, 1986b).

Despite the low rate of transmission in medical settings, the consistent use of infection control procedures to avoid the possibility of exposure to HIV appears advisable. Consistent both with the recommendations of public health officials and with the recognition that an unknown number of persons may be asymptomatic HIV carriers (Centers for Disease Control, 1988; Institute of Medicine, National Academy of Sciences, 1986a, 1986b), increasing numbers of doctors, nurses, dentists, and dental hygienists are wearing latex gloves and masks in treating all of their patients and are taking special precautions when dealing with any potentially infectious body fluid. Additional modifications in routine procedures also may be advisable. For example, in many hospitals, hypodermic needles are no longer recapped after usage but are disposed directly in specially designed containers. This change precludes the possibility of a needlestick occurring when attempting to recap the needle, thus eliminating one possible vector of viral transmission. More stringent infection control measures are necessary in settings in which exposure to blood and other infectious materials is likely to be extensive and where the potential for viral transmission is apt to be high. Many surgeons working with HIV-infected patients have begun working in multiple layers of surgical gloves and clothing in order to provide additional barriers between themselves and infectious body fluids. It is the obligation of hospitals and other health-care institutions to provide staff with the means to protect themselves from work-related HIV transmission.

Persons providing mental health care for persons with AIDS or HIV infection are generally at even lower risk for HIV infection due to patient contact than is the case with medical personnel. Nonetheless, there are mental health providers who do work in settings where exposure to blood and other potentially infectious body fluids does occur. For example, persons working in psychiatric institutions or with the developmentally disabled may find themselves in situations in which blood or other body fluids are spilled. In such cases, the infection control practices advocated for medical personnel are advisable. In most other instances, however, it is the unwarranted fear of HIV infection that is the largest barrier between health-care professionals and patients. It is to this important component that we now turn our attention.

Attitudes of Medical Personnel

Education of all persons employed in physical and mental health care settings, including administrators, doctors, nurses, orderlies, nursing aides, support staff, and janitors, is a necessary component of insuring that HIV-infected persons and those with AIDS have unrestricted access to care (e.g., Wachter, 1986). Ideally, AIDS education would be undertaken at the pre-professional level (i.e., in school or training programs) which then would be supplemented by new staff orientation. Current staff should receive training as part of work-related, in-service programs. All AIDS education must include current and accurate information on HIV transmission vectors and on means of reducing one's risk of infection in the workplace, but also should include information about risk reduction outside the work environment. Pre-employment orientation programs and the training of current staff also should emphasize the infection control policies of the institution. Moreover, because new procedures or techniques of transmission reduction are likely to be developed, training workshops to update staff must be held periodically. Anecdotal evidence indicates that training programs for health-care workers are an effective means of reducing their anxieties and, in turn, their families' anxieties about working with AIDS patients and HIV-infected persons. Such programs may facilitate the access of such persons to medical and mental health treatment programs and may reduce instances of AIDS-related discrimination in such programs (cf. Altman, 1986).

Unrestricted access to medical and mental health treatment also may be hampered by attitudes toward members of the groups at highest risk for AIDS: homosexuals and IV drug users. Although evidence of such attitudes may be less surprising among the general public (e.g., Dupree & Margo, 1988; St. Lawrence, Husfeldt, Kelly, Hood, & Smith, in press), negative attitudes toward AIDS patients, and particularly toward homosexual patients, have been documented in several studies (e.g., Kelly, St. Lawrence, Smith, Wood, & Cook, 1987a, 1987b, 1987c; St. Lawrence et al., in press). In a series of studies, Kelly and his colleagues (1987a, 1987b, 1987c) asked medical students, physicians, and nurses respectively to read vignettes about a man named Mark who was described as being either a homosexual or a heterosexual suffering from either leukemia or AIDS. After reading the vignette, participants were asked to complete questionnaires assessing prejudicial attitudes (e.g., "deserves his illness" and "dangerous to others") and willingness to interact with Mark on a social level (e.g., "attend a party where he is present" and "allow children to visit him"). All three groups of medical professionals evidenced more prejudicial attitudes toward and less willingness to engage in social interaction with Mark the AIDS patient than Mark the leukemia patient. Although physicians did not distinguish between the heterosexual and the homosexual Mark, both nurses and medical students exhibited more prejudicial attitudes and less willingness to interact socially with Mark when he was described as being homosexual than when he was described as heterosexual. Although Kelly and his associates' data do not address directly the ways in which these medical professionals might treat their own HIV-infected patients, it does not require an enormous logical leap to assume that their prejudices might affect adversely the quality of medical care administered to persons who suffered from the dual stigmas of homosexuality and AIDS.

Mental Health Care

Medical personnel are not alone in their negative attitudes toward homosexuality and gay persons. Historically, the attitudes of many mental health professionals reflect their lack of acceptance of homosexuality. For example, prior to 1973, homosexuality was included in the American Psychiatric Association's (APA) *Diagnostic and Statistical Manual (DSM)* as a mental disorder. The official view that homosexuality was a profound form of psychopathology, most recently elucidated by Socarides (1978), resulted in a belief that homosexuality could and should be "cured" through psychiatric intervention. Such "treatments" to cure homosexual individuals of their sexual orientations have included electroconvulsive therapy, hormone elevation therapy, electric shocks administered to the genitalia, emetics to induce vomiting when viewing homoerotic stimuli, and other noxious drugs (see Altman, 1971). Less aversive forms of psychotherapy, including traditional insight therapies and psychoanalysis, were often directed toward changing the sexual orientation of clients, thus returning them to "normalcy" (Coleman, 1982a). Finally, mental health workers' antipathy toward gays and bisexuals is apparent in the testimony about incipient psychopathology underlying homosexuality delivered in court cases dealing with the lives and livelihoods of these persons. For example, in 1972, Dr. Charles Socarides, a psychiatrist specializing in homosexuality, stated in a sworn deposition for a case involving the discharge of a homosexual naval civilian employee that homosexuals were mentally ill and showed symptoms that would place them between the diagnostic categories of borderline neurotic and psychotic (see Marmor, 1980).

Officially, the 1973 decision by the American Psychiatric Association's Board of Trustees to exclude homosexuality from the list of psychiatric disorders and the subsequent exclusion of homosexuality from future editions of the *DSM* were to mark an end to the designation of homosexual preference as a psychiatric condition. This exclusion was challenged by a group of psychiatrists, led by Drs. Irving Bieber and Charles Socarides, and resulted in a referendum of APA members who subsequently voted (58% to 38%) to support the exclusion (see Bayer, 1981; Marmor, 1980; Silverstein, 1985; Suppe, 1985). Although homosexuality per se was excluded from the *DSM-III* (published in 1980), a classification of "ego-dystonic homosexuality" (i.e., psychological distress and anxiety resulting from a homosexual identity) was included as a mental disorder over the protests of many prominent psychiatrists (see Bayer, 1981). However, "ego-dystonic heterosexuality" was not included in the *DSM-III* despite the arguments of numerous psychiatrists that inclusion of such a category was equally warranted (see Bayer, 1981; Marmor, 1980).

Despite official changes in classifications, many gay men and lesbians continue to report being affected negatively by attempts of psychotherapists to alter their sexual orientation, therapists' lack of understanding of the particular problems faced by gay and lesbian persons in modern society, evidence of homophobia, and the heterosexist bias that permeates psychological thought on sexual orientation (see Bullough & Bullough, 1977; Cohen & Stein, 1986; Krajeski, 1986; Morin & Charles, 1983; Nichols, 1986; Silverstein, 1985). These experiences possibly reflect the lack of training in sexual orientation issues received in most mental health curricula and a preoccupation with origins of sexual orientation (Krajeski, 1986) rather than with legitimate psychotherapeutic issues such as sexual functioning (e.g., McWhirter & Mattison, 1978; McWhirter & Mattison, 1984), the "coming out" process (Coleman, 1982b), dealing with societal homophobia, and the formation of a psychologically healthy self-concept (e.g., Cohen & Stein, 1986; Davison,

1982). Psychotherapists' negative attitudes toward homosexuality, or at best their lack of awareness of the particular issues facing gay men and lesbians, may lead them to support, explicitly or implicitly, negative societal judgments of homosexuality, thus strengthening their clients' tendencies to internalize homophobic attitudes (e.g., Cohen & Stein, 1986; Pillard, 1982; Richardson, 1987; Silverstein, 1985). Moreover, many mental health professionals continue to play the role of the inquisitor, ferreting out those persons who fail to conform to societal standards (see Moses & Hawkins, 1982; Pillard, 1982; Szasz, 1970). As a result, many gay and lesbian individuals, who otherwise might benefit from psychotherapeutic intervention, may bear resentment toward all members of the mental health profession. (See Moses & Hawkins, 1982, Sanders, 1980, and Stein & Cohen, 1986 for extensive coverage of issues related to counseling gay and lesbian persons.)

Despite the fact that, for historical reasons, gay persons who are HIV-infected or have AIDS may hesitate to seek out mental health interventions, they are likely to need psychotherapeutic interventions to cope with the psychological trauma resulting from HIV infection or AIDS (see Kübler-Ross, 1987; Martelli et al., 1987; Moffatt, 1986; Morin & Batchelor, 1984; Nichols, 1986; Peabody, 1986; Staver, 1987). Because therapeutic issues are addressed directly elsewhere in this volume, we have chosen to highlight three issues that the therapeutic community *needs* to address in order to deal effectively with the psychological components of the AIDS epidemic: (a) psychosocial factors associated with HIV-infection and AIDS and the need of professional training to deal with these issues, (b) issues of client confidentiality, and (c) professional support. These issues are highlighted briefly below.

Psychosocial Factors

Mental health practitioners, like medical practitioners, continue to be insensitive to the special needs of both HIV-infected persons and their supporting networks. One reason for this may be a lack of awareness of the needs and issues confronting those affected by the disease and an adherence to traditional notions about intimate relationships among ethnic and sexual minorities (e.g., Coimbra & Torabi, 1986/1987).

As discussed elsewhere in this volume, a diagnosis of AIDS or HIV infection results in responses similar to those associated with diagnoses of other catastrophic or fatal illnesses (e.g., Institute of Medicine, National Academy of Sciences, 1986b; Kübler-Ross, 1969, 1987; Siegal & Hoefer, 1981). Diagnosed individuals and their families may go through the traditional stages, outlined by Kübler-Ross (1969), of dealing with death and dying. However, rather than passing through these stages in an orderly fashion, the cyclical nature of the opportunistic infections characteristic of AIDS may preclude infected individuals and their families from reaching the final stage of acceptance of the fatal condition (see chapter on Therapeutic Issues for further discussion). The amelioration of an opportunistic infection, such as Pneumocystis carinii pneumonia, through medical treatment may allow patients and their families to believe that they have "licked the odds" and beaten the HIV infection itself. Such thinking permits them to return to earlier phases of Kübler-Ross's sequential stages, thus providing a temporary setback to actual acceptance of impending death.

Many psychotherapists also are unfamiliar with the particular needs of patients from the communities at highest risk for HIV infection: gay men and intravenous drug users. For example, psychotherapists' lack of awareness of the similarities and differences in the relationships of gay men and those of heterosexuals (e.g., McWhirter & Mattison, 1984; Schmitt & Kurdek, 1987), the complexities of bisexuals' relationships (e.g., Ross, 1983), and the therapeutic needs of gay men (e.g., Cohen & Stein, 1986; Krajeski, 1986) may, inadvertently, contribute to psychological distress in their clients rather than alleviating such distress. In addition, traditional assumptions about the nature of "family" and family supports within the gay/bisexual and intravenous drug-using communities may actually thwart therapists' attempts to use family members as a source of support for those affected by HIV infection and AIDS. Often, families reject their gay or IV drug-using members, either as a result of their lack of acceptance of the behaviors that define these groups or of the diagnosis of HIV infection/AIDS (cf. Moffatt, 1986; Peabody, 1986). Thus, they cannot or will not serve as a supportive network. Moreover, within the gay community, peers and friends are often more significant sources of support than are members of the traditional family unit as defined in the therapeutic literature (e.g., Morin & Batchelor, 1984; Nichols, 1986). As a result, therapists' attempts to involve the biological family may overlook what has become the "real" family for many infected persons.

Finally, psychotherapists need to be attuned to the nature of gay identity and the ways in which AIDS may affect this identity (e.g., Nichols, 1986). Many gay and bisexual men as a result of a diagnosis of AIDS or HIV infection will begin to internalize homophobia, thus resulting in greater psychological distress. Moreover, because sexuality, for some gays, is an important part of their homosexual identities (e.g., Shilts, 1987), the facts that their disease may have had its origins in their sexual activities and that such activities may have to be modified, curtailed, or ended can lead to a dissolution of a well-integrated gay identity (see Nichols, 1986). Psychotherapists need to be aware of these issues and the ways in which they can be successfully resolved.

Client Confidentiality

Therapists dealing with seropositive clients face issues of confidentiality and therapeutic trust that do not arise often with other clients. Traditionally, psychotherapists have assured clients that the issues discussed in therapy sessions are sacrosanct and that, except in extreme instances in which the therapist perceives direct harm to the client or others, information emerging in therapy is held in confidence. Indeed, many mental health professionals would insist that confidentiality is a prerequisite for successful psychotherapy. However, this becomes more complicated when doing psychotherapy with HIV-infected persons. Most pertinent are the issues that arise when an HIV-infected person involved in sexual relationships is unwilling or feels unable to convey information about antibody status to current or potential sexual partners. Because HIV is highly infectious, currently noncurable, and usually fatal, therapists may find themselves in a conflict between wishing to notify the sexual partners of the client's seropositive status and wishing to assure client confidentiality. The ideal goal in such circumstances would be to assist the seropositive individual to accept the implications of

the infection and to assist in the disclosure of the infection to partners and family members.

It is unclear how legal precedent regarding therapist-client confidentiality, such as the Tarasoff ruling in California, will affect therapists who deal with HIV-infected clients who refuse to reveal their
antibody status to sexual partners. For example, in a recent article,
Girardi, Keese, Traver, and Cooksey (1988) present arguments for
and against the culpability and liability of a fictional psychotherapist who fails to inform a client's wife of his seropositivity. The
attorneys "arguing" on behalf of the wife in this scenario propose
that the Tarasoff ruling, which requires that therapists alert potential
victims of their clients' intents to render harm, applies in the case of
this HIV-infected bisexual man because the therapist was aware that
the client had not informed his wife of his infection and was not
employing safer sex techniques. The attorneys "defending" the
therapist, who in the scenario is being sued by the now-infected
wife for liability, argue that patient confidentiality requires that the
therapist not divulge the client's seropositivity, that infection was
likely to have occurred before the therapist became aware of the
client's status, and that therefore the Tarasoff decision does not, in
fact, apply in this fictional case. The arguments presented are indicative of the complexity of the issues involved. Mental health professionals should face these issues before courts and legislators dictate
how such issues must be treated.

Professional Support

Finally, it is important to emphasize the need for psychotherapeutic support for the professionals who deal directly with persons
with AIDS or HIV infection. Staff find themselves increasingly
overburdened, and many "burn out" as a result of their efforts to
serve those clients/patients who otherwise might "fall between the
cracks" in traditional service delivery settings (e.g., Morin & Batchelor, 1984; Osborn, 1986; Wachter, 1986). As the disease
spreads, there will be increasing numbers of professionals whose
emotional and psychological resources become overtaxed, resulting
in a need for therapeutic intervention. By anticipating such needs,

mental health professionals will be better able to help the growing number of their colleagues who are affected by the epidemic.

The Economics of Health Care

The medical costs associated with the care of persons with AIDS and HIV infection are extremely high, a cost to which every U.S. household will contribute in some way. Costs will appear in a variety of forms. For example, paying patients will experience higher medical bills as physicians and hospitals attempt to recoup losses due to nonpaying patients (e.g., Meyer, 1987). There will be increases in health insurance premiums for both individuals and groups as the insurance industry attempts to minimize financial losses due to payment of claims by people with AIDS and HIV-related diseases. Finally, because many of the persons infected with HIV fall at the lower-income end of the economic spectrum, increasing amounts of public assistance will be directed toward health care, resulting, unfortunately, in higher taxes for the rest of society.

AIDS is an extraordinarily expensive syndrome to treat, with cost estimates from diagnosis to death ranging from $94,000 (Harris, 1987) to $147,000 (Institute of Medicine, National Academy of Sciences, 1986a) per patient, per year. Although costs vary from region to region, it is clear that the overall cost of the epidemic is likely to increase dramatically as the number of persons infected with HIV and those developing AIDS continues to rise. The Public Health Service estimates that the cost of treating only persons with full-blown AIDS will reach $16 billion by 1991 (Harris, 1987). The bulk of the projected costs are for direct medical expenses associated with hospital and physician costs and do not take into consideration a variety of additional expenses (e.g., payment for mental health care) that persons with AIDS and HIV-infected persons also may require. Finally, cost estimates to date do not take into account the fact that new drugs, such as AZT, will prolong the lives and, hence, the needs for health care of HIV-infected individuals. As medical advances improve, and as long as there is no actual cure for the disease, the number of opportunistic infections needing treatment and payment also will increase.

It is anticipated that an increasing proportion of the cost of AIDS will be borne by various public institutions (see chapter on Public Policy in this volume). For example, experts estimate that public and teaching hospitals, which already treat a high proportion of other indigent patients, will be asked disproportionately to bear the costs of this new group of patients (e.g., Andrulis, Beers, Bentley, & Gage, 1987; Harris, 1987; Meyer, 1987; Micheli, 1987). Similarly, as the financial reserves of persons with AIDS and their families are drained by the cost of treating the disease, governmental insurance plans such as Medicaid will be required increasingly to foot the bill for treatment. Because the budgets of both the public hospitals and the governmental insurance plans already are strained and because the prognosis for persons with AIDS is poor, medical care for these individuals is likely to suffer (Meyer, 1987). Finally, changes in governmental reimbursement programs for hospitals treating indigent patients, from allowing recovery of all costs to recovery only of costs based on the patient's Diagnostic Reimbursement Group (DRG) classification, may result in early discharge of patients with AIDS in order to minimize losses suffered by these medical institutions. As a result, concern with the costs of the epidemic may result in less adequate care for people with AIDS.

Several factors about the costs of AIDS and HIV infection are particularly important to recognize. First, health-care costs associated with AIDS, although extremely high, are only one component of the actual cost of this epidemic. Equally important are the costs associated with loss of potential productivity among infected individuals due to either their illness or death. It has been estimated that, in 1986 alone, losses in productivity due to the illness or death of persons with AIDS amounted to $7 billion, a figure that is expected to rise to $56 billion by 1991 (Harris, 1987). Second, because AIDS is considered to be a disabling condition, most persons with AIDS who have met employment requirements during their working lives will qualify for disability payments allocated to disabled persons from the Social Security Trust. Thus, as the younger working population shrinks and the number of retired workers dependent on Social Security continues to grow (in accord with demographic predictions), an additional group of even younger workers who might have paid into the Social Security system will, instead, further drain the system's financial resources.

Finally, there is the cost of AIDS to families. Families are often ill-prepared to deal with the costs associated with catastrophic illnesses and may find their financial resources strained to the limit as a result of AIDS or HIV infection. Given that persons with AIDS are more likely to be adults, a variety of outcomes are foreseeable. Adult parents of persons with AIDS may find income saved for retirement spent on their ill children, families and couples may lose their primary breadwinner or may devote all their available funds to care of the ill family member, and single individuals may find themselves financially devastated as a result of the costs of treating AIDS.

AIDS EDUCATION AND SEXUAL VALUES

Presently, education is the only vaccine we have in the fight against AIDS and HIV infection (Koop, 1987). Yet, AIDS education presents problems to many Americans. Because of the ways in which HIV infection is transmitted, AIDS education must deal with issues of sexuality, sexual behavior, and intravenous drug usage, issues that many find distasteful or embarrassing. These are not topics with which society has dealt well. For example, many are still debating the advisability of advertising condoms on radio and television, even though television depicts an extraordinary number of sexual acts nightly (e.g., Will, 1987). In many ways our discomfort with AIDS education reflects our ambivalence about sexuality in general and antipathy toward the groups, homosexuals and IV-drug users, in which the epidemic first appeared. This subsection focuses on societal responses to AIDS education efforts, especially as sexual values are reflected in such efforts. A broader discussion of AIDS education is found elsewhere in this volume (see chapter on Strategies for Education and Prevention).

AIDS Education

To date, educational programs to reduce HIV transmission have been directed largely at gay men, bisexuals, intravenous drug users, and the sexual partners of these individuals. As a result of being directed at adult populations who may be engaging in high risk behaviors, such educational endeavors have often been sexually explicit in their discussions of particular forms of behavior. These educational endeavors and the resulting furor surrounding them are discussed briefly below.

In general, sexual risk-reduction or "safer sex" programs promote a number of modes of sexual interaction that reduce or minimize the probability of HIV transmission in a sexual encounter. For example, such programs routinely advise that sexually active individuals engage only in sexual activities (such as mutual masturbation, frottage, and other forms of noninsertive sexual contact) that avoid exposure to the specific body fluids (blood and semen) known to transmit HIV. Risk reduction programs directed at gay men also often include advice about avoiding specific activities, such as "rimming" (oral-anal intercourse) and "fisting" (insertion of the hand into the rectal cavity), that are less common among heterosexuals. Moreover, persons are exhorted to reduce the number of sexual partners they have, thus reducing the probability of exposure to HIV through sexual contact. Finally, such programs also routinely advocate the use of condoms, in conjunction with spermicides containing Nonoxynol-9, to reduce the chance that persons who engage in insertive sexual intercourse will expose themselves or their partners to HIV infection. Central to the curricula of all such sexual risk-reduction programs is explicit information on routes of HIV transmission.

A variety of researchers have demonstrated that knowledge of HIV transmission routes and means of reducing exposure to HIV, i.e., "safer sex" techniques (e.g., Carter, 1986; Kelly & St. Lawrence, 1986), are correlated with modifications in high-risk sexual behaviors (e.g., Fox, Odaka, & Polk, 1986; Martin, 1986, 1987; Ostrow, Emmons, O'Brien, Joseph, & Kessler, 1986). For example, sexually explicit risk-reduction campaigns have been credited with the reduction of rates of seroconversion (e.g., Fox, Ostrow, Valdisseri, Van Raden, Vissher, & Polk, 1987; McKusick, Coates, Wiley, Morin, & Stall, 1987) and the incidence of sexually transmissible disease other than HIV infection, such as rectal gonorrhea, among gay and bisexual men (e.g., Eijrond, van den Hoek, Emsbroek, Schoonhoven, & Coutinho, 1987).

Several phenomena promulgated by risk-reduction education

programs may, either singly or jointly, account for these decreases. First, data from several studies indicate significant decreases in the number of sexual partners and the incidence of oral and anal intercourse (both insertive and receptive) among gay and bisexual men (e.g., Doll, Darrow, O'Malley, Bodecker, & Jaffe, 1987; Fox et al., 1987). Thus, behaviors that are likely to put noninfected persons at increased risk for exposure to HIV infection, if they engage in unprotected sexual intercourse with an infected individual, have been reduced. Second, these same studies have reported increases in the number of gay men and bisexuals engaging in either monogamous relationships or celibacy (e.g., Doll et al., 1987; Fox et al., 1987). Finally, condom usage among gay and bisexual men seems to have increased (e.g., Doll et al., 1987). As a result of reductions in the number of unprotected contacts with potentially infectious partners, the probability of exposure to HIV infection has been reduced in this population. The success of these educational efforts may have been enhanced by the fact that the audiences often consisted of educated and highly motivated individuals who may have had friends or associates who had AIDS or were HIV-infected.

Unfortunately, data from two studies in the United States (Fox et al., 1987; Valdiserri, Lyter, Callahan, Kingsley, & Rinaldo, 1987) indicate that barely a third of the gay and bisexual men surveyed regularly employed condoms during anal intercourse despite the fact that the vast majority knew that condoms may provide a barrier against HIV transmission. In one study, among the reasons cited for failure to use condoms were beliefs that condoms were used only by heterosexuals (26%), that they were not readily available (22%) or were embarrassing to buy (18%), and that they spoil sex (22%) or "turn off" partners (16%) (Valdiserri et al., 1987). Thus, although sexual risk-reduction campaigns have shown some success, attitudinal factors may preclude implementation of specific risk-reduction guidelines.

In addition to the individual factors that may impinge on adoption of risk-reduction behaviors, institutional concerns may discourage or forbid the use of these techniques. Although condoms and spermicides, when used jointly, are thought to inhibit HIV transmission, the use of artificial means of birth control, including condoms and spermicides, is forbidden by the Roman Catholic Church (e.g.,

Washington Post, 1987). As a consequence, controversy has arisen among the Roman Catholic hierarchy regarding *any* teaching about the use of these forms of protection in AIDS educational programs designed to be implemented in Catholic parochial schools. Three particular issues appear central in this controversy: birth control, homosexuality, and HIV transmission. Although the Roman Catholic Church insists that nonmonogamous, nonheterosexual relationships are sinful, it recognizes that transmission of HIV in either nonmonogamous or nonheterosexual relationships could be curtailed by condom usage. Thus, the Roman Catholic Church is caught between its attempts to avoid condoning homosexuality and sexual relationships outside of marriage and the prevention of further spread of the disease.

The problem facing the Roman Catholic Church is characteristic of the conflict between conservative sexual values and educational necessity that faces many public officials and private individuals with regard to AIDS education. The problems become even more complicated when the focus is education of nonadults, specifically children and adolescents. For example, the New York State Board of Regents mandated in August of 1987 that AIDS education would be a component of health education programs in all schools from kindergarten through 12th grade. However, even though the Regents made suggestions for ways in which the AIDS curricula could be implemented, it left decisions regarding content and method to the discretion of local school boards, a decision that has resulted in a great deal of controversy (e.g., "Will Regents'," 1987). As a consequence, many boards are developing curricula that stress only sexual abstinence or fail to address sexual transmission of HIV until students have reached high school when parents are less likely to object to such teachings. An example is the school board in a district with a high incidence of unwed mothers between the ages of 12 and 15 years that decided not to teach about condoms and other forms of risk-reduction behavior until students had reached the 10th grade. Fear that they would be criticized for encouraging sexual activity among their students appeared to be a primary factor influencing the development of this curriculum.

Communities in general appear to be ambivalent toward nonprocreative sexual intercourse, either within or outside of marriage.

The belief that sexual behavior should exist only for purposes of reproduction is such a central component of the Judeo-Christian ethic underlying U.S. culture that severe societal and legal sanctions have been developed historically to discourage nonreproductive sexual encounters (Paige, 1977). The fact that sales of contraceptives to nonmarried persons was restricted in some states through the 1960s, that sexual intercourse between nonmarried consenting adults remains illegal in some states, and that sex education programs still remain a subject of controversy reflect the slow progress made since Margaret Sanger was arrested for promoting contraception in the early part of this century. Yet, if we are to address effectively the AIDS epidemic, this controversy must be addressed forthrightly.

Many opponents of sex education are concerned that exposure to information about sexuality will lead to increases in sexual activity among those being educated (cf. Parker, 1982; Patton, 1987). Such concerns become central when the potential target population for education is adolescents, a group people fear will become "addicted" to sex (cf. Reiss, 1986). While the data on relationships between sexual education programs and sexual activity are sparse, *there is no evidence that indicates that exposure to sex education programs has increased the sexual activity levels of those participating in such programs* (e.g., Eisen & Zellman, 1987; Kirby, 1984; Zelnik & Kim, 1982). Adolescents who are exposed to sex education programs appear to be no different than adolescents not exposed to such programs in either their rates of sexual intercourse or their age of transition from virginity to nonvirginity (Eisen & Zellman, 1987; Kirby, 1984; Zelnik & Kim, 1982). Indeed, the transition from virginity to nonvirginity among adolescents appears to be a normal developmental phenomenon, with about 70% of teenage girls and 80% of teenage boys having had at least one coital experience (Yarber, 1987). The age at which such transitions occur appears to reflect such factors as degree of conventionality in social values, perceived control by both peers and parents, independence strivings, and engagement in non-age-normative behaviors (e.g., Jessor & Jessor, 1975). Thus, sex education programs do not promote sexual intercourse among adolescents. Rather, such programs prepare adolescents for sexual encounters by providing a working knowledge of both the mechanisms and the consequences of their sexual behavior. Beliefs that sexual education programs inevitably lead to increased sexual activity are unsupported in the research literature and should not be allowed to interfere with the implementation of AIDS education.

Although issues of curriculum content and implementation are discussed elsewhere in this volume, it is important to emphasize that the following three factors are crucial to effective AIDS education. First, the information presented must be factually accurate and current. Educators must be adequately trained, must keep abreast of developments in the research arena, and must be encouraged and have the freedom to teach all pertinent information about the disease. Second, teachers must be permitted to teach information about sexual and drug-related risk-reduction techniques. This teaching should be age-appropriate (e.g., see chapter on Strategies for Education and Prevention in this volume), but factual, risk-reduction information must be included in the education of all persons who are or may become sexually active or use IV-drugs. The importance of teaching alternatives to existing behaviors if one is to achieve behavior change is clearly demonstrated in the social learning literature (e.g., Bandura, 1969) and programs that fail to teach audiences alternatives to high-risk behaviors will not be effective. Finally, it is important that AIDS education programs strive to enhance sex-positive attitudes among those being educated. This aspect of AIDS education is covered briefly below.

Enhancing Sex Positivity in AIDS Education

Critical to the success of AIDS education efforts and, in turn, to society's success in dealing with the AIDS crisis are the values that are taught in the context of sexual education programs. The use of the term "values," however, does not mean discussions of moral, ethical, or religious premises. Rather, within this context, values refer to the emotional component of sexuality (i.e., whether one has a positive or a negative emotional response to sexuality).

The study of relationships between sexuality, affective values, and other sexually relevant variables, such as attitudes to contraceptive usage, has a fairly short history in the behavioral sciences.

Nonetheless, a variety of researchers (e.g., Caron, 1986; Carter & Caron, 1987; Fisher, Byrne, & White, 1983) have studied relationships between one particular affective response to sexuality, erotophobia-erotophilia, and a variety of sexuality-related behaviors relevant to AIDS education. According to Byrne and his colleagues (Fisher et al., 1983), erotophobic individuals are more likely to express discomfort with sexually-related information and sexual situations, to evaluate sexual situations negatively, and to show avoidance responses to sexual activities and sexually-related information. Erotophilic individuals, in contrast, are more likely to respond positively to both sexual information and to situations related to sex and sexuality. For example, in the area of contraceptive usage and comfort in discussing contraception, erotophobic individuals report that they are less likely to purchase or use contraception, and they exhibit more negative attitudes toward discussing contraception with their partners than do their erotophilic peers (e.g., Caron, 1986; Fisher et al., 1983). Thus, erotophobic individuals also may be less likely to discuss or employ safer sex practices when engaging in sexual intercourse than erotophilic individuals.

In general, erotophobia appears to have its roots in restrictive and negative socialization experiences in childhood and adolescence. For example, erotophobic individuals report more restrictive and more negative sexual socialization experiences (e.g., religious prohibitions and fear of social disapproval) than do erotophilic individuals (Fisher et al., 1983). Such experiences may lead not only to a more negative evaluation of sexuality but also to abuse in relationships. For example, Carter and Caron (1987) present data indicating that erotophobes are more likely to tolerate physical abuse in romantic relationships and to tolerate rape than are their erotophilic peers. Thus, it is clear that the values associated with sexuality are likely to have an impact on both the nature of sexual relationships and on people's willingness to take steps necessary to avoid HIV infection in sexual encounters.

The AIDS epidemic, perhaps more than any other epidemic of sexually transmissible disease, presents sexuality educators with the twin problems of alerting sexually active and potentially sexually active individuals to information regarding the sexual transmission of disease while diminishing negative affective responses to sexuality in general. Thus, it is necessary to present factual information regarding disease transmission in a fashion that does not promote erotophobia in audiences receiving such information. Rather than presenting the message that "sex is bad," sexuality educators need to convey the message that "protected sexual intercourse is good." Therefore, educational efforts may need to include information that dispels commonly held myths in populations at risk for infection (e.g., "sexual intercourse with a condom is not pleasing" or "partners who prepare for sexual intercourse are by definition sexually promiscuous" or "condoms are for contraception, not disease prevention"). In addition, educational efforts must include the clear message that, although sexual encounters increase the probability of HIV infection, such encounters are a normal, natural component of adult experience. Finally, viable alternatives (e.g., mutual masturbation) to higher-risk sexual activities may need to be offered and negative attitudes toward such activities may need to be ameliorated.

Homophobia and AIDS Education

Attitudes toward homosexuality and attitudes toward AIDS education appear inextricably intertwined in U.S. society (Frutchey, 1988). Such confusion perhaps results from the fact that AIDS first affected the homosexual community in this country, and thus it was this community that first developed educational efforts designed to slow and eventually halt the spread of the disease (Institute of Medicine, National Academy of Sciences, 1986b; Shilts, 1987). Such efforts have achieved remarkable success in addressing the spread of HIV infection and lowering the seroconversion rate (i.e., occurrence of new cases) among gay and bisexual men through the use of sexually explicit materials that clearly describe behaviors that are likely to transmit the virus. These materials have provided a model for educational efforts directed at other populations at risk for HIV infection and AIDS, such as IV drug users and their sexual partners, women, and sexually active heterosexuals.

Despite their success in reducing seroconversion rates, sexually explicit materials, especially those directed at gay/bisexual men and IV drug-users, have been the subject of controversy among politicians (e.g., Gevisser, 1987; Institute of Medicine, National Academy of Sciences, 1986b; Linebarger, 1987), newspaper columnists (e.g., Kilpatrick, 1987), and the religious community (e.g., *Washington Post*, 1987). As a result of this controversy, on October 14, 1987, the United States Senate passed an amendment (the "Helms Amendment") to an appropriations bill with a vote of 94 to 2. This amendment forbids the use of federal funds for any AIDS education, information, or prevention programs that "promote or encourage, directly or indirectly, homosexual activities" or intravenous drug usage (Gevisser, 1987). In the House, even traditional liberals voted to support the amendment and it was adopted by a vote of 368 to 47. Although health educators, including the membership of the American Public Health Association, have reacted with dismay at the passage of this amendment (e.g., Gevisser, 1987), no legislative action to date has been enacted to rescind it. Of particular concern is the fact that educational programs that have been shown to be effective in reducing or, in some cases, halting this disease will have to be reduced or eliminated.

The negative reactions of governmental agencies and politicians to sexually explicit AIDS educational efforts often are to activities less familiar to heterosexuals (activities, it should be noted, that also may be perceived as outre by many homosexuals). Most extreme have been the responses, even among many homosexuals, to an activity known as "fisting," an activity in which one individual places his entire hand in the bowel of another. Fisting was included in brochures designed for use by gay/bisexual men, not because the activity was a common one, but because it had such a high potential for resulting in HIV infection. Unfortunately, the inclusion of fisting and other activities unfamiliar to heterosexual readers (e.g., "rimming" or oral-anal intercourse, "water sports" or urophilia) may have exacerbated the misperception of homosexual activities already present in the broader heterosexual population, thus establishing homosexuals even more firmly as a group of outsiders or perverts.

Similar misconceptions have resulted from other early publicized facts about AIDS. The fact that HIV infection was most common among individuals with a high number of sexual contacts, typical of the pattern seen in any STD epidemic, reinforced the ideas that

(a) AIDS is associated with promiscuous behavior and (b) that all homosexuals are sexually promiscuous. The fact that the largest proportion of cases of AIDS and HIV infection is among the homosexual community encourages the belief that homosexuality causes AIDS or that AIDS is a plague visited upon gays by a vengeful God. The tendency to blame "victims" for their conditions fed directly into such beliefs about the nature of this epidemic while allowing heterosexuals to disregard their risk.

CONCLUSION

The AIDS epidemic offers U.S. society an opportunity to address both its homophobic tendencies and its negative attitudes toward sexuality and sexually relevant materials. The association of this disease with homosexuality has forced many Americans to come to grips with the fact that a fairly large proportion of the population is not heterosexual and, as a rising number of celebrities and associates have become infected or died of HIV-related diseases, to accept that a surprising number of individuals "passing" as heterosexuals are, in fact, homosexuals. In the process, many noninfected homosexuals have, in increasing numbers, chosen to reveal their sexual orientations to their friends and acquaintances. The fact that so many of these persons appeared "normal" prior to our recognition of their actual sexual orientations raises conflicts between our beliefs about homosexuality and the normalcy of homosexuals of our acquaintance, perhaps setting the stage for significant attitude changes about homosexuals.

Exposure to sexually explicit materials may serve to reduce the negative emotional responses to sexuality often found in segments of our society. Thus, over time, AIDS education programs may serve to desensitize the American populace to sexually-related issues and reduce anxieties about sex. The realities of the AIDS epidemic may force us, individually and institutionally, to address the sexual education needs of adolescents and others in a meaningful fashion. The frank education on sexually-related issues that this epidemic requires has the potential for reducing dramatically our cultural erotophobia. Indeed, many sexuality educators have remarked that the necessities of AIDS education have swept away previous objections to the inclusion of sexuality education programs in the nation's schools. Thus, the AIDS epidemic has the potential for addressing several sexually-related issues in U.S. society in a positive fashion.

The three issues covered in this chapter, although certainly not exhaustive of the issues that arise in this epidemic, provide some perspective on how our society has responded to the AIDS crisis and some guidance for the future. The problems created by the epidemic for individuals, families, and communities require maximum cooperation across society as a whole. Mental health professionals dealing with HIV-infected persons and persons with AIDS will need to expand their knowledge of the medical aspects of HIV infection, the medical prognosis of persons with AIDS, and the means of infection control necessary to deal effectively with the needs of clients and their families. Similarly, medical professionals will need training in the psychological concomitants of AIDS and HIV infection to meet the medical needs of their patients. Schools and other community groups need to pool their educational resources to educate not only the children in their charge but also parents and other adult family members about AIDS and HIV infection. Social service agencies, hospitals, hospices, and community health nurses will find it necessary to coordinate their efforts to provide home-based or ambulatory care for HIV-infected individuals in order to reduce the health-care costs associated with this disease. AIDS crosses traditional professional boundaries, and adequate treatment of the disease and its psychological costs will require both a multidisciplinary approach and institutional linkings that may not exist currently in all communities or states (Osborn, 1986).

Legislatures, governmental agencies, and professional organizations can do much to promote the linking of existing institutions to facilitate the needed adaptation of traditional treatment models. States in which funds normally do not pay for home health-care could modify those regulations that preclude such treatment, thus resulting in substantial savings. Professional organizations and governmental agencies could work together to plan innovative strategies that would end compartmentalization of services and make concerted efforts to insure that persons with AIDS are treated with dignity and compassion. Finally, physical and mental health professionals could develop ways in which individual members and organizations can build upon each others' strengths and skills.

Our society still must work diligently to counter hysteria about AIDS and negative attitudes associated with the disease. Professionals can do much to disseminate accurate information to affect negative attitudes toward those groups currently at greatest risk for developing the disease. Concerted efforts must be made to insure that the public receives information that is informative and accurate, but that does not unduly alarm. Such efforts will require a closer monitoring of the news media and a greater participation of scientists in reporting. Mental health professionals and health educators need to renew their efforts to reduce societal homophobia (e.g., Bryant, 1977) and remove the stigmatization of persons who are gay and of persons who have AIDS or are HIV-infected. Reduction in discrimination will do much to help persons cope with the impact of AIDS and HIV infection.

In order to cope with the costs of the epidemic, there is a need for extensive financial planning, both on the part of individuals and of agencies. Alternative modes of treatment, such as ambulatory care, may provide some financial respite, but financial costs associated with treating persons with AIDS are likely to remain high in the foreseeable future. Infected or ill individuals may find themselves avoiding needed medical care or attempting to stretch health-care dollars by, for example, reducing the prescribed amounts of medicine taken. Hospitals and other institutions may discharge individuals earlier than their medical conditions warrant in order to save costs "needlessly" spent on persons who have a fatal disease. Insurance companies may terminate the policies of persons with AIDS to save themselves and their ratepayers the cost of paying for health care of persons with AIDS or HIV infection. Financial planning is the only alternative to abandonment of persons with AIDS. Such planning needs to begin immediately.

Finally, there is a great need for psychosocial research on the ways in which individuals, families, and communities are coping with the epidemic of AIDS. The AIDS epidemic presents social scientists with a milieu in which answers to long-standing questions may be addressed. For example, our current understanding of rela-

tionships between the immune system and psychological functioning is minimal. The study of psychological functioning and general
physical health among HIV-infected persons and those with AIDS
may provide us with basic scientific information about such relationships as well as a means for enhancing the abilities of these
persons to remain healthier longer. Studies of attitude change, the
nature of familial and extrafamilial support systems, and the ways
in which families cope with the AIDS crisis may provide an extraordinary pool of information about basic psychological and social issues. Such research efforts will require the allocation of additional
funds to nonmedical research.

This chapter has presented information on several of the important issues associated with AIDS and HIV infection in an attempt to
elucidate ways in which this crisis has been and can be handled.
The AIDS epidemic presents us with a number of unique opportunities to address pressing social and interpersonal problems. By em-
bracing the very nature of the problem, the AIDS epidemic presents
us with a challenge to ignore the tendency to flee that which we
fear. AIDS forces our society to come to grips with issues that have
long been ignored or to which we have paid only lip-service. AIDS
affects all of us and the responses of our society to AIDS should
cause us to reconfirm our mutual commitments to each other as
individuals and as members of the human race. AIDS challenges
our humanity. The nature of our response may well be the basis of
history's judgment of our generation.

REFERENCES

Adkins, B. (1986). Fauci admits projected AIDS cases are speculation. *New York
    Native, 146*, 10-11.
AIDS suspicion bars surgery. (1987, July 9). *New York Times*, p. A21.
AIDS virus: Always fatal? (1987, September 8). *New York Times*, p. C1, C3.
Altman, D. (1971). *Homosexual: Oppression and liberation*. New York: Avon
    Books.
Altman, D. (1986). *AIDS in the mind of America: The social, political and psy-
    chological impact of a new epidemic*. Garden City, NY: Anchor Press.
Andrulis, D. P., Beers, V. S., Bentley, J. D., & Gage, L. S. (1987). The provi-
    sion and financing of medical care for AIDS patients in US public and private
    teaching hospitals. *Journal of the American Medical Association, 258*, 1343-
    1346.

Associated Press (1987, November 17). AIDS figure "just a guess," doctor says. *Syracuse Herald-Journal*, p. A2.

Bandura, A. (1969). *Principles of behavior modification*. New York: Holt, Rinehart, and Winston.

Barol, B., Hager, M., & Wingert, P. (1987, February 16). Koop and Bennett agree to disagree. *Newsweek*, p. 64.

Bayer, R. (1981). *Homosexuality and American psychiatry: The politics of diagnosis*. New York: Basic Books.

Boswell, J. (1980). *Christianity, social tolerance and homosexuality: Gay people in Western Europe from the beginning of the Christian era to the Fourteenth century*. Chicago: University of Chicago Press.

Broad AIDS laws signed in Illinois. (1987, September 22). *New York Times*, p. B7.

Bryant, A. (1977). *The Anita Bryant story: The survival of our nation's families and the threat of militant homosexuality*. Old Tappan, NJ: Fleming H. Revell Co.

Bullough, V. L., & Bullough, B. (1977). *Sin, sickness, and sanity: A history of sexual attitudes*. New York: Garland.

Caron, S. L. (1986). *Factors associated with contraceptive use in first year college students*. Unpublished doctoral dissertation, Syracuse University, Syracuse, NY.

Carter, D. B. (1986). AIDS and the sex therapist: "Just the facts please, Ma'am." *The Journal of Sex Research*, *22*, 403-408.

Carter, D. B. (1987, November). "Societal responses to AIDS: The real vs. the ideal responses." In S. L. Caron (Chair), *AIDS and families*. Symposium presented at the annual meetings of the National Council on Family Relations, Atlanta, GA.

Carter, D. B., & Caron, S. L. (1987). Personality correlates of attitudes toward rape and violence in late adolescence. Unpublished manuscript, Syracuse University, Syracuse, NY.

Castro, K. G., Lieb, S., Jaffe, H. W., Narkunas, J. P., Calisher, C. H., Bush, T. J., & Witte, J. J. (1988). Transmission of HIV in Belle Glade, Florida: Lessons for other communities in the United States. *Science*, *239*, 193-197.

Centers for Disease Control (1987a, August 14). Public Health Service guidelines for counseling and antibody testing to prevent HIV infection and AIDS. *Morbidity and Mortality Weekly Report*, *36*, 509-515.

Centers for Disease Control (1987b, August 14). Revision of the CDC surveillance case definition for Acquired Immune Deficiency Syndrome. *Morbidity and Mortality Weekly Report*, *36*(1S), 1-15.

Centers for Disease Control (1988, June 24). Update: Universal precautions for prevention of transmission of Human Immunodeficiency Virus, Hepatitis B virus, and other blood borne pathogens in health care settings. *Morbidity and Mortality Weekly Report*, *37*, 377-388.

Christensen, C. W., & Ringel, L. (1986). *Discrimination on the basis of sexual orientation in the state of New York.* Report of the Governor's Task Force on Gay Issues. Albany, NY: State of New York.

Cohen, C. J., & Stein, T. S. (1986). Reconceptualizing individual psychotherapy with gay men and lesbians. In T. S. Stein & C. J. Cohen (Eds.), *Contemporary perspectives on psychotherapy with lesbians and gay men* (pp. 27-56). New York: Plenum.

Coimbra, C. E. A., & Torabi, M. R. (1986/1987). Sexual behavior and AIDS in sociocultural perspective. *International Journal of Community Health Education, 3,* 269-275.

Coleman, E. (1982a). Changing approaches to the treatment of homosexuality: A review. In W. Paul, J. D. Weinrich, J. C. Gonsiorek & M. E. Hotvedt (Eds.), *Homosexuality: Social, psychological, and biological issues* (pp. 81-88). Beverly Hills, CA: Sage.

Coleman, E. (1982b). Developmental stages of the coming out process. In W. Paul, J. D. Weinrich, J. C. Gonsiorek & M. E. Hotvedt (Eds.), *Homosexuality: Social, psychological and biological issues* (pp. 149-158). Beverly Hills, CA: Sage.

Crenshaw, T. L. (1987, June 3). *AIDS.* Congressional Testimony for the Republican Leadership Task Force on Health Care, Washington, DC.

Cuomo, M. M. (August 4, 1987). *AIDS: New York's response.* Albany, NY: Office of the Governor.

d'Adesky, A. C. (1987, November 20). Antiviolence project offers support groups for survivors of heterosexist violence. *New York Native,* p. 10.

Dannemeyer, W. E. (1987, January 7). The AIDS epidemic. *Congressional Record, 133*(2), E66-E68.

Davison, G. C. (1982). Politics, ethics and therapy for homosexuality. In W. Paul, J. D. Weinrich, J. C. Gonsiorek & M. E. Hotvedt (Eds.), *Homosexuality: Social, psychological, and biological issues* (pp. 89-98). Beverly Hills, CA: Sage.

Dlugosch, G., Gold, M., & Dilley, J. (1986a). AIDS antibody testing: Evaluation and counseling. *Focus, 1*(8), 1-2.

Dlugosch, G., Gold, M., & Dilley, J. (1986b). Diagnosis/Treatment: Disclosing AIDS antibody test results. *Focus, 1*(8), 2-3.

Doll, L. S., Darrow, W., O'Malley, P., Bodecker, T., & Jaffe, H. (1987, June). *Self-reported behavioral change in homosexual men in the San Francisco City Clinic cohort.* Paper presented at the Third International Conference on AIDS, Washington, DC.

Dunne, J. R., & Lombardi, T. (1987, June). *The AIDS crisis in New York: A legislative perspective and agenda for study.* Report prepared by the staff of the New York State Senate Majority (Republican) Task Force on AIDS. Albany, NY: New York State Senate.

Dupree, J. D., & Margo, G. (1988, January). Homophobia, AIDS, and the health care professional. *Focus, 3*(2), 1-2.

Eijrond, B. D., van den Hoek, J. A., Emsbroek, J. A., Schoonhoven, R. J., & Coutinho, B. D. (1987, June). *Declining incidence of sexually transmitted diseases as a result of an AIDS education campaign*. Paper presented at the Third International Conference on AIDS, Washington, DC.

Eisen, M., & Zellman, G. L. (1987). Changes in incidence of sexual intercourse of unmarried teenagers following a community-based sex education program. *The Journal of Sex Research, 23*, 527-533.

Fischl, M. A., Richman, D. D., Grieco, M. H., Gottlieb, M. S., Volberding, P. A., Laskin, O. L., Leedom, J. M., Mildvan, D., Schooley, R., Jackson, G. G., Durack, D. T., King, D., & the AZT Collaborative Group (1987). The efficacy of azidothymidine (AZT) in the treatment of patients with AIDS and AIDS-related complex: A double-blind, placebo-controlled study. *New England Journal of Medicine, 317*, 185-191.

Fisher, W. A., Byrne, D., & White, L. A. (1983). Emotional barriers to contraception. In D. Byrne & W. A. Fisher (Eds.), *Adolescents, sex, and contraception* (pp. 207-242). Hillsdale, NJ: Erlbaum.

Foreman, J. (1986, November 21). Mass. neurosurgeon suggests quarantine for AIDS carriers. *The Boston Globe*, p. 30.

Fortunato, J. E. (1987). *AIDS: The spiritual dilemma*. San Francisco: Harper & Row.

Fox, R., Odaka, N., & Polk, B. F. (1986, June). *Antibody status and subsequent sexual activity*. Paper presented at the Second International Conference on AIDS, Paris, France.

Fox, R., Ostrow, D., Valdisseri, M., Van Raden, B., Vissher, B., & Polk, B. (1987, June). *Changes in sexual activities among participants in the Multicultural AIDS Cohort Study*. Paper presented at the Third International Conference on AIDS, Washington, DC.

Friedland, G. H., Saltzman, B. R., Rogers, M. F., Kahl, P. A., Lesser, M. L., Mayers, M. M., & Klein, R. S. (1986). Lack of transmission of HTLV-III/LAV infection to household contacts of patients with AIDS or AIDS-related complex with oral candidiasis. *New England Journal of Medicine, 314*, 344-349.

Frutchey, C. (1988). Homophobia in AIDS education: Counterproductive to prevention. *Focus, 3*(2), 3.

Gevisser, M. (1987, November 9). With friends like these . . . In response to the National March on Washington, Congress takes a swipe at gays. *New York Native, 238*, p. 13.

Ginzburg, H. M., Fleming, P. L., & Miller, K. D. (1988). Selected public health observations derived from the Multicenter AIDS Cohort Study. *Journal of Acquired Immune Deficiency Syndromes, 1*, 2-7.

Girardi, J. A., Keese, R. M., Traver, L. B., & Cooksey, D. R. (1988). Psychotherapist responsibility in notifying individuals at risk for exposure to HIV. *The Journal of Sex Research, 25*, 1-27.

Gostin, L., & Curran, W. J., (1986). The limits of compulsion in controlling AIDS. In C. Levine & J. Bermel (Eds.), *AIDS: Public health and civil liberties* (pp. 24-29). New York: Hastings Center.

Green, R. (1987). The transmission of AIDS. In H. L. Dalton, S. Burris & the

Yale Law Project (Eds.), *AIDS and the law: A guide for the public* (pp. 28-36). New Haven, CT: Yale University Press.

Hammonds, E. (1987). Race, sex and AIDS: The construction of "other". *Radical America, 20*(6), 28-37.

Harris, D. (1987, November). We'll all pay. *Money*, 109-134.

Health and Public Policy Committee of the American College of Physicians & The Infectious Diseases Society of America. (1986). Acquired immune deficiency syndrome. *Annals of Internal Medicine, 104*, 575-581.

Herald American News Service. (1987, August 30). Fear of AIDS erupts into a fire of rage. *Syracuse Herald American*, p. A1, A8.

Howe, K. R. (1988). Why mandatory screening for AIDS is a very bad idea. In C. Pierce & D. VanDeVeer (Eds.), *AIDS: Ethics and public policy* (pp. 140-149). Belmont, CA: Wadsworth.

Institute of Medicine, National Academy of Sciences. (1986a). *Confronting AIDS: Directions for public health, health care and research.* Washington, DC: National Academy Press.

Institute of Medicine, National Academy of Sciences. (1986b). *Mobilizing against AIDS: The unfinished story of a virus.* Washington, DC: National Academy Press.

Interrante, J. (1987). To have without holding: Memories of life with a person with AIDS. *Radical America, 20*(6), 55-62.

Jessor, S. L., & Jessor, R. (1975). Transition from virginity to non-virginity among youth: A social psychological study over time. *Developmental Psychology, 4*, 473-484.

Kelly, J. A., & St. Lawrence, J. S. (1986). Behavioral intervention and AIDS. *The Behavior Therapist, 9*, 121-125.

Kelly, J. A., St. Lawrence, J. S., Smith, S., Hood, H. V., & Cook, D. J. (1987a). Medical student attitudes toward AIDS. *Journal of Medical Education, 62*, 549-556.

Kelly, J. A., St. Lawrence, J. S., Smith, S., Hood, H. V., & Cook, D. J. (1987b). Stigmatization of AIDS patients by physicians. *American Journal of Public Health, 77*, 789-791.

Kelly, J. A., St. Lawrence, J. S., Smith, S., Hood, H. V., & Cook, D. J. (1987c). Nurses' attitudes toward AIDS. *Journal of Continuing Education in Nursing, 19*, 78-83.

Kilpatrick, J. J. (1987, November 16). Taxes to promote safe sodomy. *Syracuse Herald American*, p. A15.

Kirby, D. (1984). *Sexuality education: An evaluation of programs and their effects.* Santa Cruz, CA: Network Publications.

Koop, C. E. (1987). *Surgeon General's report on Acquired Immune Deficiency Syndrome.* Washington, DC: U.S. Public Health Service.

Krajeski, J. P. (1986). Psychotherapy with gay men and lesbians: A history of controversy. In T. S. Stein & C. J. Cohen (Eds.), *Contemporary perspectives on psychotherapy with lesbians and gay men* (pp. 9-26). New York: Plenum.

Krauthammer, C. (1987, October 5). AIDS hysteria: Time to cool it. *The New Republic*, pp. 18, 20.

Kreiger, N., & Appleman, R. (1986). *The politics of AIDS*. Oakland, CA: Frontline Pamphlets.

Krim, M. (1987). How *not* to control the AIDS epidemic. *The Humanist*, *47*(6), pp. 14-16, 34.

Kübler-Ross, E. (1969). *On death and dying*. New York: Collier Books.

Kübler-Ross, E. (1987). *AIDS: The ultimate challenge*. New York: Macmillan.

Lambda Legal Defense Fund. (1987). *Living with AIDS: A guide to the legal problems of people with AIDS*. New York: Lambda Legal Defense and Education Fund, Inc.

Leishman, K. (1987a, February). Heterosexuals and AIDS: The second stage of the epidemic. *The Atlantic*, pp. 39-49, 52-58.

Leishman, K. (1987b, September). AIDS and insects. *The Atlantic*, pp. 56-66, 68-72.

Linebarger, C. (1987, November 9). California Republicans label safe-sex lit. obscene. *New York Native*, *238*, p. 11.

Macklin, R. (1986). Predicting dangerousness and the public health response to AIDS. In C. Levine & J. Bermel (Eds.), *AIDS: Public health and civil liberties* (pp. 16-23). New York: Hastings Center.

Marmor, J. (1980). Epilogue: Homosexuality and the issue of mental illness. In J. Marmor (Ed.), *Homosexual behavior: A modern reappraisal* (pp. 391-402). New York: Basic Books.

Martelli, L. J., Peltz, F. D., & Messina, W. (1987). *When someone you know has AIDS: A practical guide*. New York: Crown.

Martin, J. L. (1986, June). *Sexual behavior patterns, behavior change, and occurrence of antibody to LAV/HTLV-III among New York City gay men*. Paper presented at the Second International Conference on AIDS, Paris, France.

Martin, J. L. (1987). The impact of AIDS on gay male sexual behavior patterns in New York City. *American Journal of Public Health*, *77*, 578-581.

Masters, W. H., Johnson, V. E., & Kolodny, R. C. (1988). *Crisis: Heterosexual behavior in the age of AIDS*. New York: Grove Press.

Mayo, D. (1988). AIDS, quarantines, and noncompliant positives. In C. Pierce & D. VanDeVeer (Eds.), *AIDS: Ethics and public policy* (pp. 113-123). Belmont, CA: Wadsworth.

McGrath, M., & Sutcliffe, B. (1986). Insuring profits from AIDS: The economics of an epidemic. *Radical America*, *20*(6), 9-27.

McKusick, L., Coates, T. J., Wiley, J. A., Morin, S. F., & Stall, R. (1987, June). *Prevention of HIV infection among gay and bisexual men: Two longitudinal studies*. Paper presented at the Third International Conference on AIDS, Washington, DC.

McNeil, J. J. (1988). *The church and the homosexual*. New York: Harper & Row.

McWhirter, D. P., & Mattison, A. M. (1978). The treatment of sexual dysfunction in gay male couples. *Journal of Sex & Marital Therapy*, *4*, 213-218.

McWhirter, D. P., & Mattison, A. M. (1984). *The male couple: How relationships develop.* Englewood Cliffs, NJ: Prentice-Hall.

Meyer, D. (1987, July 27). Money woes afflict AIDS hospitals. *Health Week*, pp. 6, 57.

Micheli, R. (1987, November). When AIDS hits home. *Money, 16,* 137-150.

Moffatt, B. C. (1986). *When someone you love has AIDS.* New York: Plume.

Morin, S. F., & Batchelor, W. F. (1984). Responding to the psychological crisis of AIDS. *Public Health Reports, 99,* 4-9.

Morin, S. F., & Charles, K. A. (1983). Heterosexual bias in psychotherapy. In J. Murray & P. R. Abramson (Eds.), *Bias in psychotherapy* (pp. 309-338). New York: Praeger.

Moses, A. E., & Hawkins, R. O. (1982). *Counseling lesbian women and gay men: A life-issues approach.* St. Louis, MO: C. V. Mosby.

New York Times News Service (1987, December 10). State medical colleges to fire those refusing to treat AIDS. *Syracuse Herald Journal,* p. B13.

Nichols, S. E. (1986). Psychotherapy and AIDS. In T. S. Stein & C. J. Cohen (Eds.), *Contemporary perspectives on psychotherapy with lesbians and gay men* (pp. 209-240). New York: Plenum.

Noebel, D. A., Cameron, P., & Lutton, W. C. (1987, January 19). AIDS warning: The Surgeon General's report may be hazardous to your health. *The New American, 3*(2), 25-28.

Nungesser, L. G. (1986). *Epidemic of courage: Facing AIDS in America.* New York: St. Martin's Press.

Osborn, J. E. (1986). The AIDS epidemic: Multidisciplinary trouble. *New England Journal of Medicine, 314,* 779-782.

Osborn, J. E. (1987). The AIDS epidemic: Discovery of a new disease. In H. L. Dalton, S. Burris & the Yale Law Project (Eds.), *AIDS and the law: A guide for the public* (pp. 17-27). New Haven, CT: Yale University Press.

Ostrow, D. G., Emmons, C. A., O'Brien, K., Joseph, J. G., & Kessler, R. C. (1986, June). *Magnitude and predictors of behavioral risk reduction in a cohort of homosexual men.* Paper presented at the Second International Conference on AIDS, Paris, France.

Paige, K. E. (1977). Sexual pollution: Reproductive sex taboos in American society. *Journal of Social Issues, 33*(2), 144-165.

Parker, B. (1982). Censorship threatens sexuality education. *Planned Parenthood Review, 2,* 3-4.

Patton, C. (1987). Resistance and the erotic: Reclaiming history, setting strategy as we face AIDS. *Radical America, 20*(6), 68-74.

Peabody, B. (1986). *The screaming room.* New York: Avon Books.

Pillard, R. C. (1982). Psychotherapeutic treatment for the invisible minority. In W. Paul, J. D. Weinrich, J. C. Gonsiorek & M. E. Hotvedt (Eds.), *Homosexuality: Social, psychological, and biological issues* (pp. 99-113). Beverly Hills, CA: Sage.

Reiss, I. L. (1986). *Journey into sexuality: An exploratory voyage.* Englewood Cliffs, NJ: Prentice-Hall.

Richardson, D. (1987). Recent challenges to traditional assumptions about homosexuality: Some implications for practice. *Journal of Homosexuality*, *13*(4), 1-12.

Ross, M. W. (1983). *The married homosexual man: A psychological study*. Boston: Routledge & Kegan Paul.

Rothstein, M. A. (1987). Screening workers for AIDS. In H. L. Dalton, S. Burris & the Yale AIDS Law Project (Eds.), *AIDS and the law: A guide for the public* (pp. 126-141). New Haven, CT: Yale University Press.

Sanders, D. S. (1980). A psychotherapeutic approach to homosexual men. In J. Marmor (Ed.), *Homosexual behavior: A modern reappraisal* (pp. 342-356). New York: Basic Books.

Schmitt, J. P., & Kurdek, L. A. (1987). Personality correlates of positive identity and relationship involvement in gay men. *Journal of Homosexuality*, *13*(4), 101-110.

Scroggs, R. (1983). *The New Testament and homosexuality*. Philadelphia: Fortress Press.

SerVaas, C. (1987, November). A time for forgiveness. *Saturday Evening Post*, pp. 50-55, 109-110.

Shilts, R. (1987). *And the band played on: Politics, people, and the AIDS epidemic*. New York: St. Martin's Press.

Siegal, R. L., & Hoefer, D. D. (1981). Bereavement counseling for gay individuals. *American Journal of Psychotherapy*, *35*, 517-525.

Silverstein, C. (1985). The ethical and moral implications of sexual classification: A commentary. In J. P. DeCecco (Ed.), *Gay personality and sexual labeling* (pp. 29-38). New York: Harrington Park Press.

Socarides, C. W. (1978). *Homosexuality*. New York: Jason Aronson.

St. Lawrence, J. S., Husfeldt, B. A., Kelly, J. A., Hood, H. V., & Smith, S. (in press). The stigma of AIDS: Fear of disease and prejudice toward gays. *Journal of Homosexuality*.

Staver, S. (January, 1987). AIDS: The personal side. *Facets*, 11-14.

Stein, T. S., & Cohen, C. J. (Eds., 1986). *Contemporary perspectives on psychotherapy with lesbians and gay men*. New York: Plenum.

Suppe, F. (1985). Classifying sexual disorders: The *Diagnostic and Statistical Manual of the American Psychiatric Association*. In J. P. DeCecco (Ed.), *Gay personality and sexual labeling* (pp. 9-28). New York: Harrington Park Press.

Szasz, T. S. (1970). *The manufacture of madness*. New York: Harper & Row.

Valdiserri, R. O., Lyter, D., Callahan, C., Kingsley, L., & Rinaldo, C. (1987, June). *Condom use in a cohort of gay and bisexual men*. Paper presented at the Third International Conference on AIDS, Washington, DC.

Wachter, R. M. (1986). The impact of Acquired Immune Deficiency Syndrome on medical residency training. *New England Journal of Medicine*, *314*, 177-180.

Walter, D. (1987, September 15). Congressional AIDS hearing: Gay activists now endorse voluntary testing. *The Advocate*, p. 12.

Washington Post. (1987, December 11). Bishops OK condoms as part of AIDS education. *Syracuse Post-Standard*, pp. A1, A11.

Waxman, H. A. (1987, February 10). For confidentiality in AIDS testing. *The New York Times*, p. A35.

Will, G. F. (1987, February 16). America gets 'condomized'. *Newsweek*, p. 82.

Will regents' AIDS hassle ever end? (1987, November 12). *Syracuse Herald Journal*, p. C6.

Yarber, W. L. (1987). School AIDS education: Politics, issues, and responses. *SIECUS Reports*, 15(6), 1-5.

Zelnik, M., & Kim, Y. (1982). Sex education and its association with teenage sexual activity, pregnancy and contraceptive use. *Family Planning Perspectives*, 14, 117-126.

Chapter 5

Implications for Public Policy: Towards a Pro-Family AIDS Social Policy

Elaine A. Anderson, PhD

POTENTIAL IMPACT ON AMERICAN CULTURE

The year is 2008. AIDS is a well-established epidemic whose ravages have gone far beyond those persons originally inflicted. It is a rare family which has not been personally affected by the disease. How will society deal with this crisis? Let us look at two quite different scenarios.

Scenario I

As AIDS has become a greater threat, its association with gay men and IV drug users has led to their persecution. Government has implemented repressive laws against gays, and persons suspected of

Elaine A. Anderson is Associate Professor, Department of Family and Community Development, University of Maryland, College Park, MD 20742.
Other persons who contributed significantly to this paper were: Diane Beeson, PhD, Associate Professor, Department of Sociology and Social Services, California State University at Hayward; Douglas A. Feldman, PhD, Chair, AIDS and Anthropology Task Force, American Anthropological Society; Mark R. Ginsberg, PhD, Executive Director, American Association for Marriage and Family Therapy; Carol Levine, Executive Director, Citizens Commission on AIDS for the New York City-Northern New Jersey Region; Robert M. Rice, Jr., PhD, Executive Vice-President, Family Service America; Steven M. Vincent, PhD, Psychology and Outpatient Counseling, St. Cloud Hospital, St. Cloud, MN; and Deborah Weinstein, MSW, Executive Director, Society for the Scientific Study of Sex.

drug use are imprisoned. Physical and economic survival for gay
men requires going underground and public outcries against homosexuality are common. Assaults on minorities of every sort are
prevalent, with law enforcement officers looking the other way.

Heterosexual sex has become stultified and an uncomfortable
topic for most adults. Sexual behavior is acceptable only in marriage, and persons fear divorce because it will thrust them into an
asexual life. Pregnant women who are infected with the virus are
required to have abortions and, if they become pregnant a second
time, they are sterilized. Anger expressed through acquaintance and
anonymous rape occurs in epidemic proportions. Although prostitutes are outlawed and imprisoned for life, prostitution has become
a strong underground industry, providing both an outlet for re-
pressed sexuality and the economic foundation for a strong criminal
force in American life.

Periodic testing for HIV is mandatory. Those fearing that they
have been exposed to the virus protect themselves from public disclosure through a thriving black market trade which alters records,
and they avoid all situations, such as hospitals, which might require
them to be tested. In order to escape suspicion, some infected citizens act as though they are uninfected and so risk infecting others.
Others withdraw entirely from all intimate interaction, to the confusion and dismay of those close to them. For purposes of public
health, those identified as HIV-positive are required to stay in
locked "quarantine" and to forego all physical contact with the
uninfected world. Because these centers are large and difficult to
staff, patients are left to care for themselves and each other. Because of the stigma and reduced life expectancy, only minimal
funds are allocated for health services and assignment to one of
these centers is viewed as a death sentence. To have an infected
member is a source of horror and guilt for the family, and families
either collude to protect the individual or to ostracize him/her.

Education about sex is primarily repressive and oriented to the
dangers of infection, and children are brought up to think of sex as
terrifying and harmful. As adolescents try to grapple with their sexuality, teenage suicide rates are soaring. AIDS continues to spread
throughout the society without an end in sight.

Scenario II

As the general public has learned that no quick cure is likely to stop the HIV epidemic, a new social ethic has evolved. People now recognize that their salvation from AIDS lies in their own social conscience and responsible behavior.

Early leadership was provided by the gay community which developed a process of mutual aid and care in response to their members who had contracted the disease. Accounts of the gay community's experience were reported widely by the media and noted by major social and political organizations, and their model of how to care for infected loved ones became an inspiration for the whole of society.

Drug usage is now understood as a learned response to emotional distress, and well-funded treatment programs are available to help persons learn new patterns. Families with a potential for drug dependence are identified early and given extensive therapeutic support.

Americans have come to accept joyfully the reality of their human sexuality. Parents seek to help their children understand sexuality without the ambivalent and confusing explanations used in the past. Understanding of contraception and prophylaxis is seen as essential for all, and sex education is an important and natural part of the parenting process. Parents are helped in this challenging task by a strong professional educational structure. Because of the new emphasis on contraception and responsible sexuality, the AIDS epidemic has slowed considerably.

Care of AIDS patients has required huge government expenditures. In order to accommodate these new domestic needs, the United States has had to drop its earlier emphasis upon military defense. It is now clear that the best defense is a cohesive and healthy nation that cares for its citizens and that interacts cooperatively with the rest of the world. Governmental supports for various forms of care have been developed, ranging from support for families caring for their sick members to institutional subsidies when hospitalization or hospice care is required. Private health insurance has been supplemented by universal government-supported health insurance and no one need fear that s/he cannot afford the care needed.

Because so many Americans are affected by the loss of loved ones, grief is now everyone's business. Americans turn to each other and, in the process, regain a sense of neighborhood and community. In these times of common difficulty, support groups are readily available everywhere, in industry and religious institutions as well as in social agencies.

Relationship commitment is occurring earlier and long engagements are now the fashion. Gay persons are permitted to marry and are encouraged to do so. Couples are encouraged to participate in programs designed to help them create and sustain a long and satisfying relationship. Voluntary testing for HIV antibodies is part of courtship, and testing, accompanied by professional counseling, is readily available and inexpensive. Some marriages occur even when one partner is seropositive, but this is a conscious decision made carefully by both partners. Safer sex is stringently practiced by these couples, and they rarely have children.

Easing of government restrictions has permitted the rapid development of numerous efficacious treatments, considerably prolonging the lifespan and enhancing the well-being of persons who are HIV-infected. A vaccine will soon be licensed for widespread use. Advances derived from AIDS-related research have resulted in more effective treatments for many diseases which have long frustrated the medical profession. Because of careful planning, the country can feel a sense of pride that it has been able to deal effectively with this public health crisis while improving the quality of life for everyone.

These scenarios depict two quite disparate courses. In the second, available knowledge and wisdom were used to find ways to protect, simultaneously, the health of the nation, the rights of individuals, and the quality of intimate relationships. This chapter presents recommendations geared to achieve the second scenario. It discusses those areas of public policy which must be considered if we are to achieve this goal and minimize the harmful impact of the HIV epidemic on individuals, families, and society.

THE NEED FOR A PRO-FAMILY
AIDS SOCIAL POLICY

Throughout its history the United States has had an ambivalent approach to social policy, vacillating between a belief in rugged individualism and a belief in proactive social reform. During the 1980s, many of the accomplishments brought about by the New Deal have been dismantled as government has attempted increasingly to rely on market forces to respond to social ills.

In spite of political verbiage to the contrary, there has been a lack of governmental concern about the well-being of families and, hence, a lack of governmental or bureaucratic structures which focus primarily on family needs. Many governmental programs have been developed to deal with the consequences of dysfunction in families, but rarely have these social programs been directed toward the family as a unit. Although most countries have found it difficult to establish a cohesive and comprehensive family policy, the United States lags far behind the efforts of others.

From the early years of this country, the relationship between family and government has been uneasy. Unlike most Western democracies, the Constitution of the United States does not assume protection of family life. In fact, the founding fathers chose not to mention the family in that document. The reigning philosophy of that time celebrated individualism, and the focus was on removing constraints on individual freedom. To this day, political quarrels about family policy can be traced to a conflict between concern for the individual and concern for the well-being of the family group.

Under the 10th Amendment to the United States Constitution, powers not assigned to the federal government were delegated to the various states. Issues related to family matters, such as marriage, divorce, property distribution, and child welfare, were relegated to the individual states. Thus, state laws and judicial actions, differing from state to state, created the structure that regulated families and were, in effect, the first family policies.

When state regulation failed to resolve certain family problems, the federal government was willing to step in on occasion. Government began, for example, to assume responsibility for the care of children and dependents who could not be cared for properly by their own families. However, once again, social policy emphasizing concern for the individual rather than for the total family dominated governmental activity until recent years.

By the mid-1970s, there was a small but significant press for government policy to focus more directly on the well-being of the American family and its members. American demographics were beginning to indicate that family life was changing, and many were concerned that it was being destroyed. Efforts were made to develop policies to accommodate such family trends as women's growing presence in the workplace, the need for childcare services, divorce, teenage single parenthood, and elderly dependents, as well as problems such as teenage suicide, substance abuse, and family violence. The 1980 White House Conference on Families focused attention on the relationship between government and family life, and the groundswell needed to form an American consensus on family policy was begun.

Although the 1980s have not witnessed the development of any cohesive and comprehensive family policy, political dialogue increasingly has included a discussion of the potential impact of proposed legislation on family life. Social service reform, industrial benefits, and child welfare legislation have been some of the legislative areas to consider the needs of families. The pluralism of families began to be accepted and ethnic diversity to be understood.

The assumption underlying this chapter is that the psychological and health-care issues triggered by the HIV epidemic impact directly on the family and family life. Therefore, any social policy which is developed in response to this crisis must consider also the potential implications for families and their members. In short, there is a need for an AIDS social policy which acknowledges the impact of HIV infection on human relationships and provides the supports needed by families to cope effectively with the education and care of their various members.

A DEFINITION OF FAMILY

The family, both as a social institution and a unit of affectional/ intimate expression, has a unique position within human culture. Families teach the fundamental values of bonding, belonging, and caring. Families provide socialization for their members across the lifespan, teaching for each age the values and roles important for human development.

Family, as defined in this chapter, includes both one's *family of origin*, particularly one's parents and siblings, and one's present *family of function*. The term *family of function* refers to those individuals who constitute an ongoing social and affectional intimate support network for one another. Traditionally, this network consisted of one's spouse and children (*family of procreation*) and one's family of origin. However, as the structure of the family has changed in recent years the concept of *family of function* has emerged. In the case of gay men, the functional family may include one's lover and other intimate friends. For IV drug users and prostitutes, family may include individuals in the person's life who fulfill "family-like" responsibilities. Members of one's family of function provide a broad range of emotional and material support for one another, fulfilling many of the major responsibilities and roles of the traditional family.

The responsibilities fulfilled by family are important because they provide individuals with those supports necessary for a constructive and meaningful life. There are, at least, eleven such responsibilities: (a) basic needs, including food, shelter, and clothing; (b) economic functions, including income and employment; (c) identity, including family heritage, social belonging, and personal identity; (d) affection and caring, including one's affiliation; (e) religion, including worship, prayer, and spirituality; (f) socialization, including the transmission of social values and traditions; (g) family formation and continuity, including marriage, raising children, and caring for dependents; (h) health and mental health, including health promotion and care of the sick and infirm; (i) education, including the teaching of knowledge and skills; (j) social control, including the setting of rules and norms for appropriate behavior; and (k) recreation, including entertainment and the use of leisure time.

Whether one is discussing families of origin, procreation, or function, two key principles need emphasis when discussing public policy. First, families are multigenerational units. Anything that affects an individual within a family will have an impact on others within the family, including older generations and future generations. Thus, the decisions of public policymakers will affect the physical and emotional health of the family and the larger society in both the short and the long term.

Second is the importance of maintaining open contacts among family members. Families serve their functions best when each individual in the family is able to have access to every other member, including contact between generations. Public policy on matters such as health care, psychosocial support services, education, and day care—to cite just a few of the areas affected by the HIV epidemic—can foster, limit, or cut off contact among family members. Every public policy issue must involve some clear consideration of how the various alternative policies either foster family contact or discourage such contact. To the extent that a policy maintains or facilitates such contact, the long-term health of individuals, families, and society is likely to be enhanced.

GUIDELINES FOR AIDS POLICYMAKERS

AIDS policymakers at all levels should consider the potential impact of their efforts on the ability of the family to perform successfully its vital roles and functions. Ideally, policy concerning AIDS should be designed to strengthen and protect the family's contribution rather than to debilitate or weaken it.

Because of the stigma and fear attached to the disease, its deadly physical toll, and its enormous health-care costs, policy concerning HIV-related treatment and care has a powerful potential to impact negatively on the family system, encouraging families to cast out those members stricken with the disease and generating feelings of distance and alienation among family members. Professionals concerned with the impact of AIDS and AIDS policy on family functioning must ask the following critical question: How will the proposed policy affect the ability of the family to perform its desired roles and carry out its important functions in our society?

The following principles must be remembered when assessing the potential effect of any proposed legislation on the family:

1. HIV-infected persons are not isolated individuals. They are people whose lives have implications for many other individuals and groups. Each family member, and each family unit, is a part of

a larger interactive social system. This family systemic view of society suggests that events and feelings in the life of one family member overlap and influence those of the other family members and, in turn, affect the ability of these persons to perform in other life arenas. HIV, therefore, has an impact not only on the individual and the family system but also on the broader emotional, sexual, educational, religious, political, legal, health-care, work, and economic systems with which that family and its members intersect.

2. Families should be broadly defined to include, in addition to the traditional biological and legal relationships, those committed relationships among individuals which fulfill the function of family.

3. The family may take a variety of forms. No single model of family functioning can be used to gauge the effects of AIDS policies, because no standard prototypical American family exists today. Families differ on such dimensions as religion, social class, geographic location, level of education, ethnicity, race, size, degree of intergenerational interaction, cohesion, and adaptability. Responsible strategies for rural families living with three generations under one roof, for example, may not produce desirable outcomes when applied to low-income, inner-city, single-parent families.

4. The influence of an HIV-infected family member stretches across generational and geographic boundaries and will differ as a function of role and developmental stage. The impact of the disease will depend on the status of the individual in the family and the stage of the family unit. People with AIDS may be partners, parents, children, grandparents, siblings, aunts, uncles, lovers, and, eventually, ancestors. Over time they will move from one family role to another, evolving new functions as they do so. The changing needs of individuals and families as they evolve and change over time must be reflected in policy.

5. AIDS policies should be designed to strengthen families and foster the support that families can provide. Policy development should be conducted with the intention of calling upon the positive, integrative potentials within families.

6. AIDS policy should take into account the myriad threats to the stability of the family posed by HIV infection and strive to protect and bolster family durability.

7. Families serve important and different functions depending upon where the infected member(s) is on the HIV illness-continuum. Families are important links in the chain of education and health care and should be helped to function effectively in prevention, at time of diagnosis, and during the course of the disease from asymptomatic to death.

8. The family plays a particularly important role in the prevention of HIV transmission. Families need help to teach and support HIV-preventive strategies.

9. The family's traditional role as caregiver should be fostered through policies which facilitate this role. Removing the family from this vital caregiving role, or making the cost of maintaining this role prohibitive or sacrificial to the other family members, may result in persons with AIDS becoming wards of the state or additions to the indigent homeless population.

10. AIDS policy should strive to support the functional and biological families of HIV-infected persons and persons with AIDS. In general, whenever family support is available to a person with AIDS, the plan of choice should be to foster that support with psychosocial and financial assistance. Because providing care to a loved one with AIDS can quickly deplete a family's financial and emotional resources, policies for care and treatment should augment these resources, thus enabling the family to continue to be the major source of care.

11. In addition to responsibilities, families have important rights which need to be protected, including the right to participate in decision-making regarding such issues as testing and treatment, the right to privacy and confidentiality, and the right to protection from discrimination. These rights will be discussed later in this chapter (also see Anderson et al., 1988).

Policy decisions may be made at several levels. Typically, when one thinks of policy making, *government policymakers* come to mind. These policymakers usually are at the level of federal or state officials. However, policy decisions are also made at other levels. *Communities* make policy decisions. The school board decides whether or not to allow a child with AIDS to attend school and reviews and approves the content of the courses children are taught. *Professionals* in the workplace, in agencies, and in health-care facilities make policy decisions that dramatically affect the lives of persons with AIDS and their families. *Families* make policy decisions on how they will run their daily lives, what their children will be told, how sickness is managed, and how crises are handled. Hopefully, the above principles will serve as guidelines underlying any policies regarding AIDS made at any of these levels.

SPECIFIC POLICY ISSUES

The following is a discussion of some major policy areas related to AIDS and the family. Discussion of each area is organized around the four levels of policy analysis: government, community, professional, and family. Only those levels of policy decision-making which are relevant are included in the discussion of any given policy area.

Social Science Research

In the relatively short time during which we have been aware of HIV and its linkage to the disease syndrome known as AIDS, significant research has been conducted on the biomedical aspects of the disease. Many important areas of research continue to need support (Institute of Medicine, National Academy of Sciences, 1986). The social science research needs that fall within the scope of this volume are discussed below.

Government Policy

Given the potential magnitude of the impact of HIV, epidemiologic research at a national level must be expanded. It is especially important that there be support for epidemiologic studies of the "lower-risk" populations as well as of the "high-risk/higher-incidence" groups. Data are needed on numbers of infected individuals per household or family unit and on their roles within that unit, however, such data must be collected in a way which protects the anonymity of the persons surveyed. Such efforts would facilitate the development of a more complete data base, allowing for more accurate predictions of the spread of the disease and a better understanding of the epidemiology of families and the etiologic factors involved. This could begin with baseline data collected through recommended voluntary, anonymous testing centers and through anonymous randomized samples in other settings.

An ongoing nationwide study of the epidemiology of sexual behavior needs to be established. In recent years, less and less financial support has been provided for researchers to study human sexual patterns. If we are to develop educational programs to change the sexual behaviors that contribute to the spread of HIV, we must know more about the epidemiology of these behaviors.

Understanding how HIV affects the dynamics of intimate interaction is necessary for any effective effort at education and social service support. Little research has been conducted on the interaction between HIV infection and human relationships. The extent to which such infection, or fear of infection, impedes the development of healthy intimate relationships, ranging from dating to partnering to marriage and parenting, needs to be explored. Longitudinal research from a life span perspective is needed to understand how the epidemic affects courtship and the selection of dating partners, the prevalence of extramarital affairs, and the rate of divorce. It is not yet known how disclosure of past affairs, bisexuality, or drug use affects the well-being and future of a particular marital dyad, or how HIV infection affects a couple's decisions regarding sexual behavior, birth control, and childbearing.

Research related to the psychosocial aspects of the epidemic needs to remain cognizant of the *continuum-of-care* concept important in the development of an HIV health-care system. Persons who test positive for HIV antibodies fall along an illness-continuum ranging from initial infection to death, and individuals diagnosed as having AIDS will have a different set of mental and physical health-care needs than asymptomatic individuals who have just learned that they are seropositive (see chapter on Therapeutic Issues in this volume). There should be research on the psychosocial needs of persons at different points on the infection continuum and on the needs of their families. Families may be affected in at least two major ways by HIV infection. First, their ability to fulfill the typical functions of most family units may be impaired or altered. Second, the structure and cohesion of the family may change. To be of help to families, it will be important to understand these dynamics and the variables which influence them.

Psychosocial research efforts also should be directed toward such issues as (a) the relationships among knowledge of seropositivity, disclosure or lack of disclosure of one's seropositivity, and psychological stress; (b) the psychosocial effects of HIV infection of the central nervous system; and (c) how to reduce dysfunctional societal and individual reactions to AIDS, such as scapegoating, retaliation, depression, and isolation.

Any discussion identifying prevention as a cornerstone of our current response to the HIV epidemic assumes that we have developed educational programs which produce behavior change. Additional research and development funds are needed to improve current programs and promote new ones appropriate to specific target groups. Evaluation of effectiveness, of course, should be built into all AIDS educational programs.

Finally, family impact studies should be incorporated into all research protocols related to the development of HIV-related policies. Policy recommendations regarding a wide range of issues, including health care, financing, testing, and psychosocial treatment, must be sensitive to the intended and/or unintended consequences for families.

The psychosocial effects of HIV infection on the individual and her/his loved ones are often as dramatic as the medical and need equal research attention. Such research is not only important for our understanding of human behavior, but also will facilitate the development of appropriate preventive and treatment programs for individuals and family units.

AIDS Education

Education is currently the most powerful weapon in the war against AIDS. Obstacles to the development of effective treatments and vaccines, as well as the possible discovery of additional viruses related to HIV, make it clear that prevention is essential to the public health. Dramatic reductions in unsafe practices among gay men indicate that people can and do alter their behavior when they are convinced that it is important to do so. For these reasons, an increased commitment of resources to the task of public education is strongly recommended.

Government Policy

Effective education requires federal support and funding. Only with greater commitment to education at a national level can standards be established and adequate resources be marshaled to ensure preventive education for all citizens.

In order to collect and disseminate widely the most current scientific and programmatic information about HIV and AIDS, a federal clearinghouse should be established. Equivalent to the biweekly *AIDS Surveillance Report* published by the Federal Centers for Disease Control, the clearinghouse would publish a *free* biweekly newsletter detailing the latest research findings; recently published books, pamphlets, and audio-visual resources; lists and descriptions of newly established or recently-funded research, educational, and treatment programs; and sources of available funds for evolving and ongoing programs.

A federally funded effort has been initiated by the National Institute of Mental Health to educate community health-care and human service professionals and providers. Such efforts must be carefully coordinated so as to maximize impact and must include informal caregivers, such as family members. Content must include information relevant to the caregiver's own physical and emotional health as well as to that of their patients and their families. Primary and secondary school teachers must be trained to provide appropriate sex education and health education, and monies must be made available for the development and implementation of a wide range of educational programs.

The following principles are essential to the effectiveness of education programs within a community:

Community Policy

All children have a right to be given sufficient information to enable them to protect their own health and safety. AIDS education should be placed in a context of health and sex education and be part of every school curriculum at all levels. It is imperative that children learn about AIDS within the context of a healthy understanding of sexuality, reproduction, and responsible sexual behavior. A good sex education curriculum for all children should precede education regarding AIDS and other sexually-transmitted diseases.

It is essential that such positive relationship values as love, commitment, trust, honesty, and responsible caring be emphasized. It is important, for example, that students be taught that if they become HIV-infected, they should utilize measures not to infect others. Moreover, AIDS should not be used as an excuse to erase the progress made by the "sexual evolution" during the past quarter century. Most Americans are not prepared to return to the sexual repression of an earlier era, and it is urgent that we work to safeguard the healthy advances made in our attitudes toward human sexuality.

Therefore, educational programs should carefully avoid any apparent antisexual bias and the HIV epidemic should not be used as justification for promoting such biases. Sexual repression only serves to promote the establishment of relationships in which unsafe sex may be more likely to occur, and inhibits the development of communication with potential sexual partners which facilitates the practice of safer sex.

AIDS education must be grounded in the latest social science, epidemiological, and biomedical research. Moreover, creativity and innovation will be required to develop effective educational programs, given that traditional teaching methods may not be those best suited for reaching some high-risk groups. Individuals with AIDS or ARC, and their family members, may be among the most effective educators and often are willing to share their experiences and newly gained understanding with young people. A personal connection with individuals who have AIDS, as opposed to abstract teaching materials, is especially powerful in helping people face the real issues and make the necessary, often dramatic, changes in behavior. Educational programs need to be directed toward all members of society if we are to dispel myths, quell fears, and forestall discrimination.

Family Policy

Parents should be encouraged to participate in the development and implementation of programs directed at children. Special programs designed to educate parents should be supported at local, state, and federal levels. Such programs can enable parents to be constructive forces in school programs and can help them to supplement school education with home education. The Surgeon General's mailing (Koop, 1988) to all U.S. households was an important step toward initiating informed family discussion about AIDS.

AIDS Discrimination

The United States today stands at a critical crossroad. AIDS, the disease, is only a small part of the total epidemic. Fear, lack of understanding, and bigotry have already caused at least as much disruption in the lives of affected persons as has the disease itself. The byproduct of this fear has been discrimination at virtually all levels of society against persons with, or in risk groups associated with, AIDS, ARC, or HIV infection.

For example, employers have fired employees who have, or are suspected of having, AIDS, ARC, or asymptomatic HIV infection. In addition, some employers have required employees to take the HIV antibody test. As AZT and other experimental drugs prolong the life span of persons with AIDS, the number of affected individuals in the workplace continues to climb rapidly. Although a few progressive companies have developed explicit policies protecting the rights of their employees with AIDS, most have not. It is likely that the workplace will become the most prevalent arena for AIDS-related discrimination in the near future. The National Leadership Coalition on AIDS has been an important force in helping business and industry to make responsible policy decisions regarding AIDS.

Landlords have evicted, or attempted to evict, persons with AIDS from their homes or apartments. In New York City, for example, it has been estimated that hundreds of persons with AIDS or severe ARC are homeless and forced to live in shelters, on the streets, in the subways, and in the parks. In such environments, they often become victims of multiple opportunistic infections, violence, and theft. Some landlords have refused to make repairs or provide essential services, such as heat and hot water, for tenants with AIDS. AIDS service and research organizations have been subject to discrimination on the part of unscrupulous landlords who have refused to rent office space or who have charged exorbitant rents.

Insurance companies have required a negative HIV test result as a prerequisite to insurance, have refused to cover treatment costs for persons with AIDS or severe ARC, and have terminated coverage even when the patient had no prior knowledge of his or her HIV infection. Many ambulance and ambulette drivers, physicians, psychiatrists and psychotherapists, dentists, hospital cleaning and food preparation staff, laboratory technicians, and physical therapists have refused to help or assist persons with AIDS. A survey by the Gay Men's Health Crisis in New York City found only 76 of approximately 500 funeral homes contacted by phone willing to be listed as accepting deceased persons with AIDS without charging excessive rates (Glidden, 1986).

Data suggest a dramatic increase in AIDS-related violence directed against gay men and lesbians. From 1985 to 1986, the National Gay and Lesbian Task Force documented a fourfold increase in the United States in verbal abuse, threats in which AIDS was mentioned as part of the attack, and homicides related to AIDS (*National Gay and Lesbian Task Force Newsletter*, 1987). In that one year, physical assaults against gays increased 64% and police-related activity against gays increased 72%. Even though much of the violence comes from male teenagers, no school district in the country has initiated an educational campaign specifically designed to curb this violence.

Perhaps most alarming has been the frequent discrimination against families with an HIV-infected member. Schools have resisted the admission of children with AIDS and some communities have ostracized and, on occasion, expelled such families in an effort to ensure their isolation. Parents have been loathe to disclose that the death of their adult child was due to AIDS, and remaining partners have feared that no one would wish to socialize with them. Families of caregivers have been avoided and even relatives have hesitated to visit in the family home. These varied examples point to the importance of addressing AIDS-related discrimination as it affects the family. Policies must be developed to protect families from this added stress of stigmatization which makes it difficult for them to seek needed support.

Government Policy

There is a need for an AIDS anti-discrimination policy at the national level. That policy should include the strongest possible statement against AIDS-related discrimination in every area. In order to avoid ambiguity, the policy should be highly specific, banning HIV or AIDS-related discrimination in such areas as employment, housing, prisons, hospitals, schools, nursing homes, insurance coverage, funeral homes, ambulance and ambulette services, health and mental health-care agencies, and day-care facilities. Until a national policy on AIDS is formulated, all state and municipal governments should develop their own legislation to combat AIDS-related discrimination.

State and municipal human rights commissions should develop an AIDS division that would handle only HIV or AIDS-related discrimination cases. An ombudsman should evaluate actively the patterns of discrimination in various industries and services, such as funeral homes. This cannot be done unless budgets for human rights commissions are augmented.

Community Policy

Fair housing laws should be amended to address HIV and AIDS-related discrimination. Persons with AIDS or HIV infection should not be excluded from renting or purchasing an apartment or house, nor should they be evicted from their premises. Many of these individuals are part of a functional family unit. Discriminating against the person with AIDS or HIV infection also prohibits their loved ones from obtaining suitable housing and may force a family to separate. Following the death of a person with AIDS, the family members and lovers of the deceased should not be evicted from the house or apartment. Construction of new housing for homeless persons with AIDS or HIV infection is urgently needed.

Professional Policy

Employers should be prohibited from firing, not hiring, or limiting the work of persons with AIDS or HIV infection, provided that such persons can reasonably perform the job tasks. No one should be required to take the HIV antibody test as a condition of ordinary employment, nor should the employer be allowed access to previous test results or to any record indicative that the employee has taken an HIV antibody test. AIDS education workshops should be conducted in the workplace for both management and employees. Sexual orientation or race should not be a basis for presumption of HIV seropositivity, and employment decisions should not hinge upon such considerations. The ability of persons with AIDS or HIV infection to provide for themselves economically is important for obvious reasons: being active and busy can positively affect one's mental health; many insurance policies will not cover AIDS-related illnesses and, hence, money is needed to pay the health-care bills; and, more often than not, the economic provider has members of his or her family who are economically dependent.

It is inevitable that the federal government will have to provide economic assistance through catastrophic health insurance coverage or some type of co-insurance plan, at least for persons with AIDS or severe ARC. In the meantime, health insurance companies must be prohibited from discriminating on the basis of HIV infection or risk-group membership. Insurance companies must not be allowed access at any level — governmental or health-care providers — to HIV antibody test results, and they must not be allowed to require HIV testing for enrollment purposes.

Hospitals and nursing homes should provide compassionate, nondiscriminatory care for persons with AIDS. An ombudsman at each hospital should be appointed to monitor the care of AIDS and ARC patients. Hospitals and alternate test sites should create strong linkages with existing community-based AIDS social service organizations. All human services and health-care providers, including hospitals and nursing homes, should encourage involvement by family members, lovers, and friends of the patient.

Family Policy

Although AIDS-related discrimination occurs frequently in schools, prisons, and other institutional settings, it appears most poignantly in the home. For example, the New York City Commission on Human Rights (November 1983-April 1986) reports a call from a grandmother in which she inquired where she could take the HIV antibody test. She had two children, a son whose lover had recently died of AIDS and a married daughter with two children. The mother had visited her son after the death of his lover and, subsequently, her daughter refused to allow her to visit her grandchildren because of fear they would become infected. The grandmother was heartbroken and wanted to take the HIV antibody test to prove to her daughter that it was safe for her to visit her grandchildren. Given the rampant anxiety surrounding AIDS, the family, in all its diverse forms, must be given the information and the support needed to correct such fears.

HIV Antibody Testing

The use of screening tests to identify antibodies to HIV is among the more controversial aspects of AIDS policy. There is no debate about the appropriateness of testing to screen blood donations so that contaminated units can be discarded or for purposes of identifying contaminated semen or organ donations. The controversy centers around the use of screening tests to identify infected people, either for their own benefit or for the benefit of others. Our recommendations in this area closely follow those of scientific and public health agencies (e.g., the U.S. Public Health Service). Although future developments (e.g., the availability of an effective treatment which would necessitate early detection of the disease) may justify screening on the grounds of therapeutic benefit to individuals, that is not true at present.

Government Policy

We support the position of the U.S. Public Health Service, the Surgeon General, and the National Academy of Sciences, among others, that mandatory (i.e., legally required) HIV screening to obtain marriage licenses, for admission to hospitals, at drug treatment centers, at sexually-transmitted disease clinics, for employment, or for other social benefits or entitlements is not warranted at this time. The use of screening tests by the military, the Foreign Service, and the Labor Department's Job Corps has already been instituted by the federal government and there is little point in discussion of these in this chapter.

The arguments against mandatory screening are both reasoned and prudent: (a) mandatory screening would be an invasion of privacy that would not be balanced by public health benefits; (b) many of the high-risk populations, fearing further discrimination, would seek to avoid being tested; (c) there would be a high likelihood of false negatives due to the unpredictable lag between time of infection and development of antibodies; (d) there would be a high number of false positives in populations with a low reservoir of infection, with ensuing unnecessary emotional distress; (e) scarce resources would be diverted from programs and populations where these funds could have a more potentially powerful impact on the spread of the disease; (f) there are too few trained counselors to provide the necessary pre- and post-test counseling; and (g) there are currently too few well-established laboratories to handle the volume with sufficient accuracy and no federal guidelines to regulate these. Moreover, if massive mandatory screening were to become the law, the confidentiality required to prevent human rights violation, especially in the areas of employment and insurance, could not possibly be safeguarded by states and municipalities.

At the same time, it is recognized that voluntary testing, as an adjunct to sensitive counseling and with informed consent, can help some infected people to accept the reality of their infection and motivate them to modify their behavior so as to protect themselves from re-exposure and to protect others from becoming infected. Therefore, the widespread availability of voluntary testing, preceded and followed by counseling, is recommended, either under

conditions of anonymity or with strict confidentiality protections. It
is important that the counseling staff be well trained in the psychosocial implications of both positive and negative test results, and
that they be skilled in facilitating couple and family communication
at times of extreme stress. Where possible, it is recommended that
those who are tested bring with them to the pre- and post-test counseling sessions a friend or relative who can provide necessary support.

Community Policy

Agencies that provide services to people whose behavior might
put them at risk for HIV infection (e.g., drug users, gay men, adolescents, sexual partners of drug users, and women in their childbearing years) should incorporate education about testing and make
appropriate referrals. Voluntariness, confidentiality, and pre- and
post-test counseling should be essential characteristics of any testing program. More readily available well-staffed HIV testing centers are needed throughout the United States to provide free, easily
scheduled, voluntary, anonymous testing with appropriate pre- and
post-test counseling to all who wish to utilize this service.

There is no medical or compelling public health reason for routine screening of school children. The issues concerning screening
for foster-care and day-care children are discussed below in this
chapter (see section on Children).

Professional Policy

Physicians and other health-care and social-service workers who
believe that an individual with whom they have a professional relationship may be infected, or may be at risk of becoming infected,
should counsel that person about risk and offer him or her the option
of being tested. Testing should never be done without an individual's consent. When testing is being considered for infants or children, consent should be obtained from their parents or guardians, as
in other matters of health care. If individuals decline to be tested,
they should be counseled to behave as if they were infected. If they
agree to be tested and are seronegative, they should be counseled on
ways to avoid becoming infected and reminded about the possible

advisability of later retesting. Testing should be routinely available in health-care settings in which there is a high likelihood that clients will be infected. However, because of the ramifications of a positive test result, taking the HIV antibody test should never be treated as "just another medical test."

Family Policy

The decision to be tested is an individual one, but it is also one that involves other family members, especially sexual partners. Individual autonomy and privacy must be balanced by obligations to others. Partners should be encouraged, and facilitated, to have an honest and open discussion about the pros and cons of testing, and resources must be readily available to help them deal with the test results (see chapters on Treatment Issues and Societal Implications in this volume for more discussion on HIV testing). Couple and family therapy can be a valuable tool in reaching decisions about testing as well as in coping with the results.

Health Care for HIV and Related Illnesses

The need for effective delivery of health services to HIV-infected persons and persons with AIDS or ARC presents health-care policymakers in both the public and private sectors with compelling and difficult challenges. Providing health care to an increasingly debilitated, chronic population with a limited life expectancy is an enormously complex task, unprecedented in its capacity to tax our existing system. The issues involved include access to and the appropriate delivery of care and treatment; the recruitment of sufficient well-trained health-care personnel; the provision of adequate numbers of beds in hospitals, long-term care facilities, and other settings; and the challenge of financing this care.

Community Policy

It is crucial that the rights, privacy, and dignity of HIV-infected persons and persons with AIDS and their families be respected in all treatment settings at all times. This overarching principle must always be preserved.

Two other principles also should be remembered. First, care and treatment must be provided from a multidisciplinary biopsychoso-cial perspective. Second, to be effective and efficient, care for HIV-infected persons and persons with AIDS must be integrated among the various health-care programs funded and administered at the local, state, federal, and private-sector levels. Comprehensive inte-grated medical and psychological care for the patient and the family must be present at all levels of service delivery, including the outpa-tient clinic, the acute-care hospital, home health care, the extended-care facility, and hospice care. At every stage of the illness, a "sys-temic" focus must be preserved.

There is an inherent interrelationship between the necessity for care and treatment for HIV-infected persons/persons with AIDS and the necessity to provide adequate funding to support this care. The mental and physical health care provided will be determined by available funds. The funds that are made available will be deter-mined, at least in part, by the need for care and treatment. These issues are clearly circular. However, it is vital that the service re-quirements dictate the available funding rather than the reverse. It would be catastrophic if services were determined primarily by the funds that were available. Thus, a discussion of health-care financ-ing for HIV-related illnesses should start with the question of what social and medical services are needed. This inductive approach to policy formation ultimately will best serve the public interest.

Professional Policy

To the extent possible, a network of services for HIV-infected persons, persons with AIDS, and their families should be developed and integrated within the established health-care delivery system. This integrated service delivery must combine the latest biomedical information with an understanding of and sensitivity toward the psychological sequelae of HIV infection. An integrated care system should be staffed by trained personnel at every level of the delivery structure, from clerical and support staff to medical staff. They should not only understand the complexities of HIV infection but also be committed to integrate biomedical treatment with psychoso-cial concerns. One example of a viable conceptual model comes from the burgeoning field of family systems medicine, which integrates the biomedical and the psychosocial with an appreciation for the needs of a family within the context of systems theory. That is, HIV-infected persons and persons with AIDS are viewed not in isolation from their environment but rather as active participants influenced by and contributing to the many "subsystems" with which they interact. Another appropriate example is hospice care which integrates the treatment necessary to comfort the chronically ill, respect for the dignity of the individual patient, and involvement of the individual's family in the treatment program.

Care and treatment of HIV-infected persons and persons with AIDS should take place in the least restrictive and most appropriate setting. Continuum-of-care should be part of any service delivery plan, including outpatient treatment, partial hospitalization, acute-care inpatient settings, after-care facilities, home health care, chronic and long-term care, and hospice care. HIV-related care must be easily available in a variety of geographic locations.

Many services for HIV-infected persons and persons with AIDS can be included in outpatient settings. However, as the illness progresses, the continuum of care must advance to an increasingly acute and then chronic level. In the years ahead, it is inevitable that many thousands of persons with AIDS will be in need of such care. A service delivery structure must be planned now if it is to be in place when a large percentage of the estimated 1.5 million HIV-positive Americans manifest AIDS-related symptoms. Because families are likely to be the site of care for many AIDS patients, we must work now to enable families to provide appropriate care (see Watkins et al., 1988, for the report of the Presidential Commission on the Human Immunodeficiency Virus Epidemic). This challenge is a major imperative to which the health policy community must respond.

Government Policy

Governments at the local, state, federal, and international level must develop a significantly expanded and targeted health-care delivery system for the care and treatment of HIV-infected persons and persons with AIDS. This system must be coordinated with existing health resources in communities, be attentive to biomedical developments, and be sensitive to the psychosocial needs of HIV-infected persons, persons with AIDS, and their families, including the rights of privacy and confidentiality. The thrust of government-derived health and social policy should be to provide universal access to necessary health services, with regard for the appropriate level of care within a continuum of care. This help should be provided in a nondiscriminatory manner and not be based on one's ability to pay. Thus, a partnership among business, labor, and government, both the private and public sectors, must be formed to ensure that adequate care and treatment are provided.

Considerable discussion and creativity will be entailed in designing an equitable system with sufficient funds to allow for both the development and implementation of programs. Whichever treatment strategies are selected, they must be appropriate for the various populations at risk for HIV infection, including gay men, IV drug users and their partners, hemophiliacs and their partners, children, and non-monogamous heterosexuals.

Children

Policies concerning children with AIDS are particularly complex. All children, by virtue of their age, are dependent and vulnerable. Their parents are presumed to be the natural protectors of their interests. When parents are unable or unwilling to assume this role, others (e.g., relatives, court-appointed guardians, and social service agencies) must step in. Children at risk of contracting AIDS are in jeopardy in several ways. In the case of perinatal transmission, the mother is, by definition, infected. If she is not already ill, she is at risk of developing symptoms and, eventually, dying.

Currently, most cases of perinatal transmission occur in Black and Hispanic mothers (Rogers, 1987). HIV-infected women from these groups are often either IV drug users or the sexual partners of IV drug users. They already bear the burden of discrimination and poverty even without the added weight of HIV infection. Furthermore, in many cases, the birth of an infected baby is often the first sign that the mother is infected and that HIV already may be a threat to family stability. A baby born under these circumstances — infected, perhaps ill, the unwelcome herald of illness in the family, and a member of a group already suffering severe social discrimination — has a poor chance in life.

Articulation of the policy issues surrounding children is still on the horizon. Increasing numbers of children and their families will be affected by policy decisions not yet made. All such decisions must take into account the material and emotional needs of children; the importance of maintaining, wherever possible, a family structure that can support these needs; and adequate social and community services to support the families.

Government Policy

At the federal level, sufficient levels of funding should be channeled through state and local agencies to provide needed services. Federal officials also can play a part in reducing fear and stigma by educating the general public about the lack of evidence for casual transmission and the importance of accepting children with AIDS, ARC, or HIV infection into schools and other community settings.

State agencies and city and local governments can play a similar role. They are directly responsible for education, foster-care, day-care, and health-care policies that will affect children and their families. These policies will have to juggle the needs of infected children and their families, the concerns of workers who provide services, and the other funding needs in the community. Local circumstances will dictate specific policies. However, all policies should be designed to fulfill society's obligations to children.

Community Policy

Many of the most important policy decisions will occur at the local level. In terms of school attendance, the American Academy of Pediatrics, the U.S. Public Health Service, and the *Surgeon General's Report on Acquired Immune Deficiency Syndrome* stress that casual contact between infected children and their schoolmates is not a risk for the transmission of HIV. The Surgeon General's report states, "None of the identified cases of AIDS in the United States are known or are suspected to have been transmitted from one child to another in school, day care, or foster care settings" (U.S. Public Health Service, 1986, pp.23-24).

No blanket rules can be made for all school boards to cover all possible cases of children with AIDS, and each case should be considered separately, as would be done with any child with a special problem, such as cerebral palsy or asthma. A good team to make such decisions jointly with the school board would consist of the child's parents, a family physician, and a public health official (Committee on Infectious Diseases, American Academy of Pediatrics, 1983).

Attendance at day care and placement in foster care present more problems, because infants and preschool-age children do not have the same ability to control behavior and bodily excretions that elementary school-age children do. However, with adequate staff education and precautions, these children ordinarily can be placed in such settings (Committee on Infectious Diseases, American Academy of Pediatrics, 1987). Here, too, individualized decision making is central.

Because day care is not a legal right, and because most day care is offered through private institutions and individuals, it is particularly important that governmental agencies monitor the policies of these agencies to make certain that children with AIDS, ARC, or HIV infection are not systematically excluded.

Two problems demand particular attention: confidentiality and consent for testing. Because information about a child's serostatus can have potentially devastating consequences if it becomes known to people other than those who have direct responsibility for the child, special care must be taken to protect confidentiality. The question of who has a legitimate need to know this information must be discussed thoroughly and carefully with special attention to the particular circumstances. All those who are deemed to have a need to know also must be made aware of their responsibility to keep this information confidential.

Testing for entry to day care raises other issues. Adults ordinarily have the opportunity to give voluntary, informed consent for their own HIV antibody testing. This process includes information about the test and interpretation of the results, whether they are negative or positive. Parents and guardians should have the same opportunity to give consent for a child, or to decline testing, as long as they understand fully the reasons why the test may be considered appropriate. Counseling is essential not only for adults who are being tested, but also for those bearing the responsibility for a child's welfare.

Another aspect of consent is the question of whether foster parents should have information about a child's serostatus before they agree to take the child. Practice in this area is divided. Some agencies refuse to screen children or to divulge this information to prospective foster parents, whereas others will do so upon request. It is understandable that foster parents might wish to have this information, both in planning appropriate child-care and in deciding whether to commit their personal resources to a particular child. However, policies should be constructed in ways that will give potential foster parents complete information about risks and outcomes and, at the same time, not discourage them unduly from taking on this responsibility. The issue of liability for a foster care agency must also be considered. Children with AIDS, ARC, or HIV infection are particularly dependent on foster care because frequently one or both parents are also ill and unable to care for them. Family care of some form should not be closed to them by virtue of their infection.

If it is impossible to place some children with AIDS, ARC, or HIV infection in foster care, day care, or schools, appropriate alternative facilities must be devised to give such children as normal an existence as possible. However, alternate facilities should not be considered the first choice for placement. It is important that these children have the opportunity to experience as normal a life as they are able to tolerate physically.

Professional Policy

Professional education and training must include information about pediatric AIDS, ARC, and HIV infection and the most up-to-date treatment and research protocols. Education is particularly important for health-care, day-care, and education staff who will have direct contact with infected children. The risk of becoming infected through working with these children is small but does exist. Workers must be trained in appropriate infection control measures and prepared for the extraordinary stress of dealing with infected, termi-

nally-ill children. Persons who have had experience in pediatric on-
cology may be able to provide advice to staff involved in developing appropriate stress-reduction and anti-burnout programs.

Family Policy

All members of a family are affected when a child has AIDS,
ARC, or HIV infection. The birth of such a baby may place severe
strain on a marriage or other relationship. Uninfected siblings also
may suffer deprivation and stigmatization, and may worry about
their own health or that of their mother or father. The family focus
on the infected child may alter family dynamics and functioning.
Family members should be made aware of these far-reaching effects. Professional family therapy should be available to assist families in adjusting to the situation and in providing the best care for
all members of the family.

Women

AIDS affects women in many ways. Women are related to, work
with, and care for persons with AIDS. They are family members,
friends, lovers, and colleagues of persons with AIDS. Women may
become HIV-infected themselves and, therefore, capable of transmitting the disease to their lovers, partners, and unborn children.
Policies concerning women and AIDS should reflect the total array
of women's needs for education, health care, and services, and not
focus solely on their potential for infection and transmission.

Special attention must be paid to women's reproductive roles and
rights. Given the high risk, currently estimated to approach 50%,
that an infected pregnant woman will bear an infected infant, prevention of infection in women must be given a high priority at all governmental, professional, and community levels. Women must receive
information about their risks and the ways and means to protect themselves from infection whether that involves access to condoms or
support for abstinence. Pregnant women must be given explicit opportunities for voluntary and confidential or anonymous testing and
compassionate counseling regarding their options should they be seropositive.

Policies that promote AIDS prevention must take into account the varied cultural, religious, and personal values affecting a woman's decision to become pregnant and to bear a potentially infected child. The possible models for counseling fall on a continuum from purposeful lack of advice to coercion. Genetic counseling supports choice and is, theoretically, a value-free presentation of the risks. The public health model is more directive, emphasizing prevention of perinatal transmission. Given the degree of invasion of body and privacy that would be entailed, forced abortion or sterilization of infected women is not an acceptable policy option.

Policy options should preserve voluntariness and choice but should not shrink from presenting the medical and social realities of AIDS. Alternatives to pregnancy, such as job and education, should be encouraged and funded for those infected women who choose to avoid pregnancy or to exercise their legal right to abortion.

Risk Reduction

Membership in a risk group does not cause AIDS. *Risk behaviors do*. An HIV-negative male couple who have been in an exclusively monogamous relationship for the past 10 years and who do not inject drugs are not at risk for AIDS. A teenage girl who forgets to use her condom and spermicide several times may be at risk for AIDS, depending on the history of her partners. Not who one is, but what one does creates the problem.

Government Policy

The U.S. Department of Education should take the lead in providing and funding a massive AIDS risk-reduction program directed specifically at the various sociocultural subpopulations throughout the United States. Condoms, spermicides, and literature on AIDS and HIV infection should be made available at no cost or on a sliding-fee scale upon request. Television, radio, newspapers, magazines, and other media should be utilized. The messages should be easily understandable, explicit, and not moralistic. It is the responsibility of the federal government, in concert with state and local officials, to educate the American public about HIV infection and AIDS. Punitive measures, such as quarantine, mandatory HIV antibody testing, and travel restrictions, will only drive persons most at risk for HIV infection underground. Efforts must be made to reduce the stigma of AIDS, not to enhance it.

Community Policy

The specific needs of those groups who have been most affected must be addressed. Efforts should be made to enhance the dignity of the millions of gay men around the world, and families of gay men should be encouraged to be emotionally supportive of them. State and municipal governments should actively seek to put an end to AIDS-related discrimination. Society should be supportive of two gay men who choose to live together in a committed monogamous relationship. It must also be recognized that monogamy is not for everyone and that conscientious safer sex practices with more than one partner is a lower risk alternative than not practicing safer sex with one infected partner.

Prostitution will not be stopped by AIDS, but its risks can be minimized. Prostitutes should be encouraged to use condoms and spermicides during vaginal intercourse and to refrain from anal sex. Legalization of prostitution would permit greater regulation of the practice and, in turn, increase safety both for prostitutes and their clients.

Drug rehabilitation centers and methadone programs must be established to meet the demand for treatment of intravenous drug users. For those who cannot stop shooting drugs or who lack the desire to stop, needles and syringes should be distributed to terminate the practice of sharing "works." "Shooting galleries," gathering places where drug users congregate to share drugs, should be closed throughout the United States. Intravenous drug users must become better informed about disinfectant practices. More important, the social conditions that lead to IV drug use — unemployment, illiteracy, poverty, racial discrimination, inadequate housing, and dysfunctional family life — must be addressed and corrected.

Persons who are in jails and prisons also are at higher risk for HIV infection, and policies to promote safety for infected and non-infected prisoners and staff must be instituted. Many prison inmates are members of families to which they will return. Enhancing health care and safety, as well as the availability of counseling for incarcerated individuals, will enhance and protect the future well-being of their family members. Condom distribution in jails and prisons, along with safer sex information, may protect the health of many individuals, including their families and the society to which many will return. Increased opportunities for conjugal visits may help to decrease the frequency of high-risk sexual behaviors.

Professional Policy

Voluntary HIV testing should be encouraged for (a) individuals who are not practicing safer sex techniques at all times and who have not been in an exclusively monogamous relationship for at least a decade; (b) persons who have injected drugs or have been sexually involved with individuals who have done so; (c) individuals who received a blood transfusion or blood products between 1979 and Spring, 1985; (d) women who wish to have a child and whose history places them at risk of HIV infection; and (e) persons for whom lack of knowledge about their serostatus has become a source of high anxiety. It is absolutely essential that HIV testing be anonymous or confidential. A "confidential" HIV test result that is recorded on the named individual's computerized medical file at a hospital, clinic, physician's office, or laboratory is *not* confidential.

It is important that blood and blood products continue to be carefully screened for HIV and other related viruses. Because a large percentage of hemophiliacs became infected before blood screening and heat treatment of Factor VIII were introduced, support services for them and their families are necessary. Within this population, infected adolescent hemophiliacs need special attention. Not only do these adolescents have to cope with their potentially life-threatening health condition, but they also have to handle normal adolescent sexuality concerns while being fully aware of their infectious status.

All risk-reduction efforts should consider the welfare of the entire family system, including lovers, and these persons should be involved in risk-reduction education simultaneously with the particular at-risk or infected individual. Social service agencies and educational institutions must have funds available to implement the extensive risk-reduction programs which are required and, hence, a well-planned and well-developed financing mechanism must be implemented immediately.

Financing of Health-Care Delivery

Decisions regarding funding for a health-care delivery system to assist HIV-infected persons, persons with AIDS, and their families must be based on service delivery needs, not on available funds. This principle is particularly important for an AIDS health-care delivery system, where the needs quickly will exceed the available resources. Extending national health benefits for catastrophic coverage regardless of age should be considered. Such an extension would reduce the likelihood that many persons with AIDS or severe ARC will face destitution if inadequately insured. The broadest solution to the financing question lies in some form of national health insurance. The model for financing discussed in this chapter is but one among many alternatives.

Government Policy

The best system for financing the care and treatment of HIV-infected persons, persons with AIDS, and their families would seem to be a partnership between the private sector (principally through employer-based health benefit programs) and government funding. It is increasingly evident that the costs of providing necessary care and treatment for persons with AIDS is extraordinarily high. AIDS, a long-term illness, requires substantial, recurring, labor-intensive, long-term care. In combination, these factors are very costly. It is likely that the expense of care and treatment for persons with AIDS will become a significant drain on our private-sector health benefit plans, on the government, and even on our entire economy. For example, Scitovsky and Rice (1987) have estimated that the direct costs of providing health care to persons with AIDS rose from $630 million in 1985 to over $1.1 billion in 1986. The direct costs will continue to rise, so that by 1991 they will exceed $8.5 billion. Economists have estimated that by 1991, aside from the staggering medical costs of the illness, the HIV epidemic will have cost our nation over $55 billion in lost personal income and other such factors. Now is the time for both private industry and government to design financing projects that will provide necessary funds at the required fiscal levels.

Private-sector health benefit plans, whenever available, should provide coverage for HIV-infected persons and persons with AIDS, but this cannot be the exclusive coverage. Ten to 15 percent of the U.S. population — 37 million Americans — are covered by individual and small-group insurance plans; another 37 million have no health insurance at all (Arno, 1987). These two groups represent a disproportionate number of persons at high risk for AIDS. Intravenous drug users often are uninsured, and many members of the gay male community are self-employed and therefore more likely to be enrolled in individual or small group plans and subject to stricter underwriting criteria. Health benefit plans should not discriminate against persons with AIDS or HIV infection by denying or limiting coverage. Rather, private sector plans must continue to provide coverage to the limits of their allowed benefit structures, with the federal government providing a re-insurance or "stop-loss" form of back-up protection. In the partnership that is envisioned here, the government would invest in the care and treatment of persons with AIDS and HIV infection, yet not assume the entire financial burden for these services. Some policymakers are suggesting that there be a federally mandated "tax" on health benefit premiums to provide funds to assist with the financing of needed services for persons with AIDS and ARC. Consideration should be given to this idea, with appropriate regard for the rights, privacy, and dignity of persons with AIDS and ARC. It may be a viable approach to the issue of financing.

Catastrophic health coverage is designed to insure an individual and his or her family against serious and costly events beyond their control, events such as a serious illness requiring lengthy hospitalization and long-term care. This is the situation with AIDS. It is recommended that a system of catastrophic care coverage be developed which includes persons with AIDS or ARC. The system envisioned would be parallel to the hospice program, a system of care for terminally ill patients affirmed by Congress in recent years and now included within the benefit structure of Medicare. However, a health-care financing program for persons with AIDS need not be included within Medicare. This is only one *possible* structure.

Other structures should be considered by the Congress, the federal Health Care Financing Administration, and other governmental institutions.

Recognizing that many HIV-infected persons do not have health insurance, the federal government, in partnership with private industry and local and state governments, should initiate and fund a "means tested voucher-type system" for persons with AIDS or ARC to use in paying for their health care. Assuming that treatment protocols will become increasingly standardized and that the number of experimental procedures will increase, persons with AIDS or HIV infection must remain free to choose from whom and where they wish to receive health-care services. With a voucher system, a person with AIDS or ARC could take his or her benefit to any government-sanctioned treatment setting.

In this model, a person with AIDS or ARC who was privately insured would first need to use and exhaust all benefits provided through his or her own private health benefits program. It is possible that the government would, in an as yet undetermined manner, assist by subsidizing such care. This would be the "means test" component of the program: the use of available benefits. In addition, there should be some mechanism for co-payment by an individual who has sufficient resources to afford a reasonable co-payment. However, if it becomes a deterrent or barrier to care and treatment, we do not recommend that a co-payment provision become a part of any means test.

Therefore, the central part of a program to finance care and treatment for HIV-infected persons and persons with AIDS would be coordinated and funded heavily by the federal government, with some assistance from both state and local governments. The most effective system might be one in which the federal government would develop and then apply a series of criteria for the different levels of care within an appropriate continuum-of-care setting providing health-related services for persons with AIDS or HIV infection. At each level of a continuum of care, appropriate criteria would be developed. This process must involve input from all of the relevant constituencies, including both consumers (persons with AIDS or HIV infection and their families) and health-care providers. Care for HIV-infected persons and persons with AIDS must be integrated within the established health-care delivery system. Standards must be developed to guarantee that those settings providing care to HIV infected persons and persons with AIDS have the facilities and staff available to provide necessary services of the very highest quality. A national network may evolve of those service delivery settings that have met federally sanctioned criteria to provide care and treatment to HIV-infected persons and persons with AIDS. It is probable that most of the needed facilities already exist. These extant facilities can be combined with newly developed facilities to form the federally sanctioned, but not federally administered or directly controlled, settings. This plan is parallel to the federal approval program which qualifies hospitals to receive reimbursement from the Medicare program.

Such a system would be expensive to develop and administer. It would, however, provide a framework for a collaborative system of care that could be positioned over the next few years to meet the needs of HIV-infected persons and persons with AIDS. It would allow for universal access to care. There are, however, problems with the design. First, a bureaucratic superstructure must be created. Second, this type of reimbursement structure would be complex, with funding based on chronicity and factors relevant to actual costs of care at different developmental stages of the virus. Moreover, given the size and complexity of such a structure, confidentiality would be difficult, but not impossible, to maintain. Further, this model might, unintentionally, create a network of AIDS and HIV infection treatment centers that would suffer from discrimination of many types.

Despite these possible criticisms, it is a fundamental responsibility of government to assure the availability of and access to necessary and appropriate health-care services. The model described above provides a vehicle for the federal government to fulfill its responsibility of providing needed health-care services for HIV-infected persons and persons with AIDS. Neither private industry nor government alone can carry the burden.

Finally, sufficient fiscal resources must be made available by federal and state government, together with private-sector services, to fund necessary research, education, and training. Therefore, funds must be made available to continue basic and applied research, including both biomedical and psychosocial research, with appropriate attention to social and behavioral science. It would be a tragic error for social and behavioral science research to be sacrificed in favor of biomedical research. Both perspectives of inquiry are necessary.

Funding for education and training must include targeted efforts directed at three groups: (a) individuals at high risk; (b) professionals who may become involved with the care and treatment of HIV-infected persons, persons with AIDS, and their families; and (c) the general public. Educational and training efforts must be systematically developed and well funded. Prevention, through the reduction or elimination of high-risk behaviors, could slow the spread of the epidemic. Proper education and training is our best chance at prevention. These tasks collectively—research, education, and training—must be funded through both existing programs of support and newly developed programs. Funds must come from both the public and private sectors.

SUMMARY RECOMMENDATIONS

The following summarize the primary family policy recommendations discussed in each of the above sections of this chapter:

Research

- Maintain ongoing studies of HIV epidemiology, including low-risk groups, and of numbers and roles of family members infected.
- Establish an ongoing nationwide study of the epidemiology of sexual behavior.
- Establish research to investigate the interaction between HIV infection and changes in relationship and family development.
- Develop longitudinal research with a life-span focus.
- Incorporate family impact analysis into all research related to AIDS policy development.

Education

- Mount a federally coordinated and funded effort to educate health and human service professionals, lay providers, families of HIV-infected persons and persons with AIDS, persons at highest risk for HIV infection, and the general public about HIV infection, modes of transmission, and impact on physical and emotional health.
- Provide a good sex education curriculum for all children prior to AIDS education.
- Develop educational programs that enable parents to be involved in the sex/AIDS education of their children.

Discrimination

- Develop a national policy against HIV and AIDS discrimination.
- Develop fair housing laws to protect HIV-infected persons, persons with AIDS, and their families.
- Conduct AIDS education workshops in the workplace for both management and employees.
- Reduce the likelihood of intra-family discrimination by educating about the non-risk of casual contact.

HIV Testing

- Provide readily available anonymous voluntary HIV testing, or testing with strict confidentiality protections, preceded and followed by individual counseling, and, when appropriate, couple and family therapy.
- Agencies who work with groups at risk (e.g., drug users, persons with STDs, women in childbearing years, and adolescents) should provide education about and referrals to HIV testing.
- When HIV testing is being considered for infants or children, consent should be obtained from their parents or guardians. Counseling should be provided regarding how to avoid HIV-infection and ways to prevent transmission if infected.

Health Care for HIV Infection and Related Illnesses

- A significantly expanded and targeted health-care delivery system for care and treatment of HIV-infected persons, persons with AIDS, and their families must be developed.
- Treatment should be based on a continuum-of-care model and be provided at multiple levels of service delivery such as the family unit, the outpatient clinic, the acute care hospital, the extended care facility, and the hospice.
- Treatment should be based on an integrated biopsychosocial model, and include both biomedical and psychosocial care for HIV-infected persons, persons with AIDS, and their families.

Children

- Educate the public regarding the safety of admitting HIV-infected children and children with AIDS into schools and day-care centers. Governmental agencies should monitor the policies of agencies to make sure that such children are not systematically excluded.
- Educate staff about the necessary precautions to be taken by guardians of HIV-infected children and children with AIDS in foster care and by the staff of day-care settings.
- Develop alternative facilities for HIV-infected children and children with AIDS who are too ill to be placed in foster care, day care, or school.
- Develop stress reduction techniques for professionals who work with children with AIDS.
- Provide family therapy to families who are the caregivers for HIV-infected children and children with AIDS.

Women

- Educate women about ways to protect themselves from HIV infection and the relationship between HIV infection and pregnancy.
- Provide pregnant women the opportunity for HIV testing and related counseling.

Risk Reduction

- The U.S. Department of Education should fund a massive HIV risk-reduction program directed at various sociocultural subpopulations.
- Develop more drug rehabilitation centers and methadone programs; expand the number of clean needle programs; and reduce the social problems experienced by many drug users, such as unemployment, inadequate housing, and family stress.
- Enhance HIV risk-reduction and counseling opportunities for incarcerated individuals so as to protect both them and the families to whom many will return.
- Develop educational and support services for HIV-infected hemophiliacs and their families, with special attention given to adolescent hemophiliacs.

Financing of Health-Care Delivery

- Develop a federal system of catastrophic care coverage to supplement private benefit structures.
- Develop a network of service delivery settings that have met federally sanctioned criteria for the care and treatment of HIV-infected persons and persons with AIDS. Such federally sanctioned criteria should be developed with input from HIV-infected persons, persons with AIDS, their families, and health-care providers.
- Provide sufficient levels of funding for research, education, and training.

REFERENCES

Anderson, E. A., Beeson, D., Feldman, D. A., Ginsberg, M. R., Levine, C., Rice, R.M., Vincent, S. M., & Weinstein, D. (1988). AIDS public policy: Implications for families. *New England Journal of Public Policy, 4*(1), 411-427.

Arno, P. S. (1987, June). *Private health insurance and the AIDS epidemic: Distributing the economic burden.* Paper presented at the annual meeting of the Association for Health Services Research, Chicago, IL.

Committee on Infectious Diseases, American Academy of Pediatrics. (1983). School attendance of children and adolescents infected with Human T-Lymphotropic Virus Type III/Lymphadenopathy-Associated Virus. *Pediatrics*, *72*(3), 430-432.

Committee on Infectious Diseases, American Academy of Pediatrics. (1987). Health guidelines for the attendance in day-care and foster-care settings of children infected with Human Immune Deficiency Virus. *Pediatrics*, *79*(3), 466-469.

Glidden, K. (1986). *Funeral home resource list survey*. New York: Gay Men's Health Crisis.

Institute of Medicine/National Academy of Sciences. (1986). *Confronting AIDS: Directions for public health, health care, and research*. Washington, DC: National Academy Press.

Koop, C. E. (1988). *Understanding AIDS*. Washington, DC: U.S. Public Health Service.

National Gay and Lesbian Task Force Newsletter. (1987). Washington, DC: National Gay and Lesbian Task Force.

New York City Commission on Human Rights. (November 1983-April 1986). *Report on discrimination against people with AIDS*, pp. 1-47.

Rogers, M. T. (1987). AIDS in children: Report of the Centers for Disease Control National Surveillance, 1982-1985. *Pediatrics*, *79*(6), 1008-1014.

Scitovsky, A. A., & Rice, D. P. (1987). Estimates of the direct and indirect costs of Acquired Immunodeficiency Syndrome in the United States, 1985, 1986, and 1991. *Public Health Reports*, *102*(1), 5.

U.S. Public Health Service. (1986). *Surgeon General's report on Acquired Immune Deficiency Syndrome*. Washington, DC: U.S. Public Health Service.

Watkins, J. D. et al. (1988). *Report of the Presidential Commission on the Human Immunodeficiency Virus Epidemic*. (Write: Presidential Commission, 655 15th Street NW, Suite 901, Washington, DC 20005.)

Epilogue —
AIDS:
Opportunity for Humanity

Marvin B. Sussman, PhD

An epilogue is a message after everyone else has said their part. In one sense, it is a view from on high. The creator of the epilogue views what has occurred from a multi-faceted perspective, reflects on it, and pontificates about the future. The intent is to analyze events, to raise questions, and to provoke new thoughts and further critiques.

CHAOS AND ACTION

Cataclysmic, terrifying, and emotionally-moving events evoke action at the highest governmental levels. Beginning with policy statements or edicts, officials engage in actions usually resulting in temporary solutions. Such ameliorations are unlikely to reach the root of the problem.

Once it was recognized that AIDS was a crisis reaching beyond the Gay community (eons of time after the first pleas were made in the late 1970s), dramatic action was initiated. A President's AIDS Commission was formed. After months of wrangling and the resignations of some Commission members, a report was released in June, 1988, with nearly 600 recommendations designed to prevent further spread of the virus, provide care for those who are HIV-infected, and promote biomedical research to establish a cure (see Watkins et al., 1988). Primary attention was given to the 1986 estimate by the Centers for Disease Control that up to 1.5 million peo-

Marvin B. Sussman is Emeritus Unidel Professor of Human Behavior, Department of Individual and Family Studies, University of Delaware, Newark, DE 19716.

ple may be infected. The data necessary to sustain, reject, or modify this estimate will come from a pilot study in three large cities establishing the feasibility of a national random household blood-testing program and routine testing of blood from patients at hospitals and clinics in 30 metropolitan areas.

In addition to commissions, studies and reports, monies in increasing amounts have become available for distribution to eager takers. Almost any idea for research on the virus or for treatment or for educational programs is supported. There is a "birthquake" of activity, mostly well intentioned, with ameliorative and temporary outcomes rationalized as worthwhile. The consciousness of governmental elites is being raised and the entrepreneurial juices are beginning to flow.

Tremendous personal gain is possible, especially when activities are couched as efforts to control the epidemic. Other-orientedness is blended with self-interest and the opportunity to become a hero or heroine. It is a situation where all may benefit, except perhaps the person with AIDS. The political and economic advantages to be had from involvement in AIDS policies and programs should not be underestimated. Persons with AIDS, family members, and friends are voters, and their concerns will have significant impact. As the epidemic spreads to the heterosexual population, political activities are heightening. Members of the legislative and administrative branches of state and federal governments scurry to initiate prevention programs and to allocate emergency funds to stem the epidemic and to treat those infected by the virus. Their actions are swift, filled with a sense of urgency and commitment, especially in those instances where a well-loved family member or friend has contracted AIDS. Numerous political protectors of society's immune system are arising and will use the AIDS panepidemic to their particular advantage. One can anticipate that the platforms of all political parties will contain provisions to exorcise the demon AIDS, hopefully the virus and not the host.

NEEDED:
NEW PARADIGMS FOR WORLD COOPERATION

The World Health Organization has reported an increasing incidence of AIDS in over 120 countries. Malcolm Parks, President of the

Family Health International, indicates that "AIDS . . . remain[s] the most significant new disease to appear since the rise of scientific medicine" (Editorial, *People*, 1987, p. 2). Forecasters do not see the eradication of this dreaded disease in this century or in the first decades of the 21st century. Yet, the approaches to handling this crisis are, for the most part, unilateral. Although there is increasing cooperation, particularly among scientific groups, the approach in most societies, including the United States, has been to erect barriers, holding to the view that AIDS is *somebody else's problem*. It is an import and, as a consequence, the legal, political, and ethical issues and solutions are not as relevant as the issues of control.

The power and suddenness of the spread of HIV has terrorized populations and raised the basic question, "Why is the human immunological system — the basic system for survival of humankind — breaking down around the world?" Could it be that individual immune systems are breaking down because world and national systems are collapsing? Could the breakdown of the worldwide immune system simply be a reflection of the breakdown in nature's immune system, a spin-off of the rapid destruction of the environment? A shadow appears to be cast upon all the world, requiring new paradigms of global integration in order to save our Earth. AIDS may be just the impetus needed to achieve this necessary cooperation. It is a crisis so formidable that it will require all the nations of the world to work together to eradicate it. New visions of world organizations and superordinate international goals will be necessary, extending well beyond the problems presented by AIDS.

PLAGUES AND THE BREAKDOWN OF HUMAN VALUES

Plagues and epidemics have existed throughout human history. In the modern period, syphilis and gonorrhea were considered to be of epidemic proportions, at least in the United States. In medieval times, the bubonic plague wiped out a substantial portion of the population of Europe, and laws, statutes, and practices were instituted having both deleterious and positive effects on succeeding populations. Let us assume that the current AIDS crisis reaches epidemic proportions, and that it is identified by ruling elites to be a plague. A plague is defined as a situation in which current institutions are incapable of controlling a disease, there are few promising methods to prevent its occurrence or to treat it successfully, and the numbers of infected people are increasing at such a high rate that families and other institutions are unable to cope with the resulting problems.

Associated with the labeling of a disease as a plague is considerable misinformation about its causes. Segments of the population may be blamed as the prime sources of infection and drastic measures subsequently taken to segregate these populations from the mainstream of their respective societies. Acting primarily out of fear and verbalizing a desire to protect the common good, draconic solutions may be offered. In a recent "Dear Abby" letter, a reader from Cocoa Beach, Florida, suggested that AIDS "victims" (reader's usage) be branded so that everyone could be forewarned not to have sex with that individual. The reader did not insist that the person be branded with a hot iron, as done to cattle. A tatoo or bracelet mandated by statute would be sufficient. Abby, with more than conventional wisdom, replied, "AIDS is an incurable disease—not a crime. And your suggestion is inhumane and in itself a crime against the dignity of humanity" (Abby, 1988, p. 46). If AIDS comes to be viewed as a plague by modern societies, a large proportion of the population may support some type of demarcation of infected populations.

Plagues and epidemics have both negative and positive consequences. The many possible scenarios resulting from the HIV epidemic are yet to be written. One possible negative scenario would be the segregation of those who have the disease from those who do not. Whether this occurs depends at least partially upon the extensity and intensity of the disease and whether the particular individuals are seen as infected through their own actions or the actions of others. Individuals who do not share needles as part of their drug use, or are not involved in prostitution, or do not engage in sexual practices conducive to the spread of the virus would be less likely to be ostracized and, in turn, segregated.

James Curran and his colleagues, in their study of the epidemiology of HIV infection and AIDS in the United States, report that there is a disproportionate number of cases among Hispanics, Blacks, drug users, their sex partners, and their infants. They say that the "relative risks of AIDS for Blacks and Hispanics are two to ten times as high in the northeast as in other regions of the country because of the concentration of IV drug abuse-related AIDS" (Curran et al., 1988, p. 610). The available data, according to current estimates, indicate that, because a large number of Americans are already infected, morbidity and mortality will continue to increase in the foreseeable future, especially among young and middle-aged men in Black and Hispanic minorities where there are large numbers of IV drug users already HIV-infected. If the incidence of the disease continues to rise at the current rate, and if there is only limited success in the cure or prevention of the disease, it is possible that efforts will be made to segregate portions of these populations, using legally enforced edicts and police measures.

Wholesale segregation, blaming of selected populations, and widespread pogroms characterized the experiences of many people during the Middle Ages as a consequence of the Black Death, the bubonic plague epidemic which swept through Europe from Asia in the middle of the 14th century (Swenson, 1988). Events of the past seem to repeat themselves in regular patterns, as if little learning in the art of being human has occurred. Fear and self-righteous blaming of minorities and the poor is a concomitant to any widespread plague or epidemic.

Denial and blame go hand-in-hand. The ruling elites, usually the upper-middle and professional classes of a society, initially indicate that what is occurring is not their problem but one of the untutored, uncleaned, and nonreligious groups. Swenson (1988) indicates there was extensive denial during the cholera and influenza epidemics occurring in the United States in the 19th and 20th centuries. One also can make a strong case that there was an AIDS denial in this country in the early 1980s when the first cases were diagnosed and brought to the attention of the authorities. It was several years and many deaths before AIDS was recognized as a problem not only for those infected but for the whole of society.

Blaming a group for causing a disease is a common phenomenon associated with plagues and epidemics. It has been common to refer to AIDS as either the "Haitian disease" or the "homosexual disease." We still talk about the Asian flu. Swenson (1988) reports that outbreaks of influenza in the United States and Western Europe in the early part of the 20th century resulted initially in high levels of denial among the western countries and derogatory exchanges among the nations. The French referred to the epidemic as "the Spanish Lady" and the Spanish referred to the influenza as "the French disease." The matter did not stop with such derogatories made at teas and cocktail parties or in disguised diplomatic messages. In a number of European countries infected by the Black Death, the Jews were blamed for causing the disease by poisoning the wells and, as a consequence, thousands of them were burned at the stake. For centuries, prostitutes have been blamed for causing epidemics, such as cholera, by passing it on to their "clients." Even today, in the face of great efforts at disease control by legalized prostitution, prostitutes are viewed as the conduits of AIDS and no amount of empirical evidence to the contrary is likely to change this popular view of the world's oldest profession (Swenson, 1988).

The consequences of blaming are determined largely by the extent to which the blamers are organized. Letters to editors and occasional newspaper reports or stories are relatively ineffectual. However, when a constituted minority or lobby group begins a series of actions castigating or blaming the victims for the disease and its actual or potential consequences, they may have some impact. There is a growing propensity to blame those with AIDS for their own infection. A number of religious groups believe that persons with AIDS are receiving retribution for their immoral behaviors. This type of discrimination must be monitored closely to prevent radical acts that go beyond endemic stigmatization. If the incidence of AIDS increases among religious functionaries who potentially will be spearheading this movement of "justice" and retribution, the fervor of the blameless may be neutralized. During the Black Death, the effects upon the Catholic church and clergy were drastic. Over half of the priesthood died in the plague. Although this consequence did not deter burning Jews at the stake, it turned a large number of individuals away from the church and reinforced the growing Protestant movement.

CONFLICTS WITHIN THE SCIENTIFIC COMMUNITY

For almost five years, there was a patent conflict between the Pasteur Institute in Paris and the U.S. Department of Health and Human Services over who invented the AIDS antibody test-kit assay. It took the President of the United States, Ronald Reagan, and the French Prime Minister, Jacques Chirac, to effect a settlement in March of 1987. This high-level political settlement basically recognized Robert Gallo of the National Cancer Institute and his colleagues and Luc Montagnier at the Pasteur Institute and his associates as joint inventors, thus terminating the many legal maneuvers which were threatening to tear apart the international research community (Barnes, 1987). Less obvious were the reasons for this conflict: economic gain and professional recognition (i.e., becoming a modern-day hero with a supportive myth not unlike Percivale's search for the Holy Grail). Conflicts within the scientific community, with high stakes in professional reputation and economic return, are not unusual. As incidence rates have increased, AIDS has been forced "out of the closet" and attracted the attention of vested-interest groups and the media. It has become apparent that there is no unified, holistic, well-thought-out plan for research and treatment but rather a scrambling approach among professionals and scientists for new discoveries, new fame, and, perhaps, a Nobel prize. These conflicts, no doubt, will continue into the 21st century — a sad legacy indeed!

One illustration of the intensity of such conflict is the debate between the biologist, Peter Duesberg, and Robert Gallo, David Baltimore, Anthony Fauci, Malcolm Martin, and other AIDS researchers over whether HIV is sufficiently virulent to cause AIDS. Dr. Duesberg, a member of the National Academy of Sciences and credited for doing creative and pioneering work in the field of virology and cancer-causing genes during the 1970s, is requesting evidence that a virus labeled HIV has caused a breakdown of the immunological system. Professor Duesberg has taken the position, "Not only is HIV too inactive to cause AIDS . . . HIV acts like no known virus because of its long latency and . . . it persists despite the production of antibodies" (Booth, 1988, p. 1487). Duesberg's search for absolute proof is unlikely to end soon, given that he finds correlations unacceptable in establishing HIV as the etiological agent in AIDS.

The ultimate consequences of these professional jealousies and conflicts for those with AIDS and their families remain unknown. The intensity of these professional debates and conflicts is unlikely to abate until substantial progress is made in obtaining a vaccine and effective treatment protocols, thus curtailing the incidence of the disease and alleviating its destructive effect.

AIDS AND ITS IMPACT ON FAMILIES

AIDS attacks the economic well-being of families and drains their relationships, resources, and psychic, spiritual, and social energies. Under existing government policies, the onset of a chronic illness and ensuing disability requires that individuals and their families pay for a substantial share of the care costs. Only when families are economically depleted are they entitled to government health-care programs such as Medicaid. If the individual has health insurance, payment from this third-party source is possible, but often it is contingent upon the individual continuing to work. Most individuals who lose employment also lose their health insurance coverage.

Given the lifetime estimates of the cost of care required by an AIDS sufferer, it is obvious that the family will continue to share an increasingly high economic burden. The Presidential Commission (Watkins et al., 1988) has estimated that annual treatment costs for a person with AIDS are approximately $40,000 and that the costs for provision of medical care to the anticipated 173,000 persons with AIDS in 1991 will be approximately $8.5 billion (or 1.4% of U.S. personal health care expenditures). As drugs and other treatment procedures become more available and effective, thus prolonging the life of AIDS patients, an increase in maintenance costs is expected. These figures do not include the loss of earning power and potential contribution to the family's and the nation's economic resources. Nor do they take into account the draining of resources from other health care needs.

One can anticipate that insurance companies, currently paying for the care of persons with AIDS under policies which were designed to provide some support for long-term illness and disability, are likely to change their present procedures and to advocate testing insurance applicants for seropositivity. This will diminish further the number of persons with AIDS eligible for insurance reimbursement and place increased burdens on their families for support and on public institutions for long-term health-care programs. Given these realities, it is clear that AIDS will require a fairly dramatic transformation of current policies and practices regarding long-term health care. The health care of the entire nation is at stake, and creative action is called for that will ensure the well-being of the next generation of families.

One of the most obvious social effects of AIDS is the current trend toward the extended one-partner relationship, a trend that is likely to increase in incidence in the coming years. There has been a downward shift in the rate of extramarital sex, reflecting a lifestyle change for many marital partners as more and more practice sexual monogamy. There is, however, no reason to believe that the "sexual revolution" has played itself out or that we are going back to a Victorian mentality, full of sexual myths and inhibitions. Rather, AIDS has shifted the sexual pattern from swinging or having sex with multiple partners to a concentration on better sex with a single partner. This should in no way diminish the recognition and enjoyment of sexuality. Current educational programs that urge safer-sex techniques during lovemaking assume that many individuals cannot tell at this point in time whether or not their partners are carrying the AIDS virus. However, once it is established that one's current sexual partner does not have the virus, it is possible for the couple to engage in sexual activities of any type, without worry.

It is predicted that families, however described or identified, will be the main support system for the family member with AIDS. Increasingly, they will assume the burden of providing not only the economic support but also the care for the infected individual throughout the various stages of treatment. The psychic impact of watching a relatively young person deteriorate, responsible for loving and compassionate care yet helpless to reverse his/her condition, has yet to be established. The stress surrounding the uncertainty of the disease, the complications of treatment, the in-and-out-of-hospital episodes, and the stigma and discrimination experienced by many caretakers is yet to be studied and understood. On the other hand, the giving of one's self that is required can lead to profound spiritual growth. It is necessary to tap one's deepest, most mature, humane self and, in turn, to recognize the spiritual qualities and emotional needs of the person with AIDS. The care and treatment of the family member with AIDS will be, for some, a transforming experience resulting in deepened consciousness and a commitment to serve. For others, it may leave emotional scar tissue, resulting in a need for therapy and costly rehabilitation.

The heavy emotional cost of care will force policymakers, legislators, and human service organizations to identify those individuals who relate well to persons with AIDS and to use family members, however defined, as allies in the treatment process. New paradigms of care, and an evolution in human values, hopefully will unite families, friends, human service professionals, volunteers, and other committed persons in a common service to provide the hope, care, and love required by persons with AIDS as they fight for survival and prepare for death.

Families of persons with AIDS experience social stigma and isolation, fears of contagion and infection, guilt, anger, grief, and economic hardship (Macklin, 1988). From this suffering of heart, mind, and soul may emerge a mythic structure focusing on healing not only the ills of the specific individual but also the ills of our modern culture. AIDS then would become, by its very devastation, the harbinger of a new humanity in which the immune systems of all individuals, all societies, and all of nature would be nourished, cared for, and protected. A necessary transformation from "me as self" to "we as unity" would occur and, in turn, the whole system would change. Families—recharged by the AIDS crisis—may well be the catalysts and the models for this crucial transformation.

REFERENCES

Abby. (1988, January 27). Reader proposes the branding of AIDS victims just to be safe. *Wilmington News Journal*, p. 46.

Barnes, D. M. (1987, April). AIDS patent dispute settled. *Science*, *236*, 17.

Booth, W. (1988, March 25). A rebel without a cause of AIDS. *Science*, *239*, 1485-1488.

Curran, J. W., Jaffee, H. W., Hardy, A. M., Morgan, W. M., Selik, R. M., & Dondero, T. J. (1988, February 5). Epidemiology of HIV infection and AIDS in the United States. *Science*, *239*, 610-616.

Editorial. (1987). AIDS in perspective. *People*, *14*(4), p. 2.

Institute of Medicine, National Academy of Sciences. (1986). *Confronting AIDS: Directions for public health care and research*. Washington, DC: National Academy Press.

Macklin, E. (1988). AIDS: Implications for families. *Family Relations*, *37*(2), 141-149.

Swenson, R. M. (1988, Spring). Plagues, history, and AIDS. *The American Scholar*, *57*(2), 183-200.

Watkins, J. D. et al. (1988). *Report of the Presidential Commission on the Human Immunodeficiency Virus Epidemic*. (Write: 655 15th St. N.W., Suite 901, Washington, DC 20005.)

AIDS:
Sources of Knowledge
for the Seeker

Kris Jeter, PhD

"Rumors spread faster than AIDS" was the theme of a 1988 public service television announcement. One cause for the runaway rumors appears to be the variety of printed matter published on the Acquired Immunodeficiency Syndrome. Individuals from varied walks of life, ranging from faith healers to physicians, sensationalists to scientists, liberals to conservatives, atheists to the religious, have decided to "jump onto the bandwagon" to write their thesis on AIDS. Each has a view to be published. Each has a dollar to make.

After the Jim Jones Guyana killings in 1979, a book on his cult was written and published in 2 weeks. This rapid turnaround time from one mind to the potentiality of many minds has found its heyday in the subject matter of AIDS. The dissemination of medical research findings, social supports, and political strategies can mean the difference between life and death and, hence, urgency is warranted. Yet, the professional in family studies, bombarded with a mass of available literature, may ask, "What are the critical books on AIDS? Which writings are exemplary and constitute a basic body of knowledge?"

In this analytic essay I shall review some selected books, audiovisuals, and articles on AIDS. Some of the books were recommended by Jim Holmes, the Coordinator for Information Services, The Gay Men's Health Crisis Center in New York City. Other

Kris Jeter is Director, Programs and Communication, The Possible Society, 800 Paper Mill Road, Newark, DE 19711.

241

sources I gleaned from my search in bookstores, health centers, and libraries.

I write this fully aware of the impact of AIDS on my own life. Although the press has tended to sensationalize AIDS on its front pages, the obituaries usually neglect to indicate when death was due to an opportunistic infection associated with AIDS, such as Pneumocystis carinii pneumonia (PCP), cytomegalovirus (CMV), Mycobacterium avium-intracellulare (MAI), Candida, herpes simplex, cryptococcal meningitis, toxoplasmosis, or cryptosporidiosis. I suspect that Bob, a friend and "Big Man on Campus" of my undergraduate days, died of a cancer associated with AIDS. I thank Bob for his sincere companionship. I know that Leonce, the pianist and physician who assisted my mother through her dying process, died of an AIDS-related cancer. I remember him and his family with love and respect. I think of my co-worker, Ron, a professor with the diagnosis of AIDS, and his partner, Chuck, a computer specialist with the diagnosis of ARC (AIDS-Related Complex). I support them in their will to live and think of them often with love. And, I contemplate the persons with the diagnosis of AIDS whom I do not know personally. I applaud the young man who, anticipating his own death, embroidered a square in his memory for the National Names Project/AIDS Quilt on display in Washington, D.C. in October, 1987. I acknowledge others and their families and friends who embroider their golden dreams and actual lives. This essay is written to honor their influence on my life and on the course of society.

HISTORY

In 1985, Allan M. Brandt, Assistant Professor of the History of Medicine and Science at Harvard Medical School and Harvard University, wrote *No Magic Bullet: A Social History of Venereal Disease in the United States Since 1880*. In 1987, he expanded the text to discuss AIDS.

In Victorian times, the middle-class family became the norm. Married couples lived in separate homes and devoted themselves to the rearing of children. This concept of the family was threatened in the mid-20th century by the rise of divorce, female education, late age of first marriage, increased costs of householding, and decreased number of children.

Gonorrhea and syphilis were thought to sterilize women and to be transmitted through childbirth to the newborn. Physicians treated patients with mercury, 180 degree Fahrenheit hot water retrojection, and potassium iodides. They spoke out against premarital and extramarital sexual relations. Between 1899 and 1913, eugenic marriage laws were passed in seven states and medical examination of all prospective bridegrooms was required. Fear spread. Foreigners were considered to have wanton sexual behaviors and to be the source of all prostitution. The Immigration Act of 1891 prohibited entrance into the United States of persons with a communicable disease. In the name of preservation of the family, social hygienists promoted sex education while physicians and social reformers campaigned against prostitution. Broadway plays, discourses on white slavery, monographs of vice commissions, public relations campaigns, and courses in sex education expressed the sentiments of the social hygiene movement.

In 1905, German researchers isolated the cause of syphilis and, the next year, August Wassermann invented the diagnostic test for syphilis. In 1909, Nobel laureate immunologist, Paul Ehrlich, discovered Salvarsan, the first effective remedy for syphilis. He said that "the antibodies are magic bullets, which find their targets by themselves" (Brandt, 1987). From that time on, researchers and physicians, patients and laypeople craved the magic bullet for whatever the particular malady.

Historically, venereal disease wounded more soldiers than any other disease and yet its debilitating effects were ignored. For example, almost 20% of U.S. Civil War soldiers became infected with gonorrhea and syphilis. However, until the Wassermann test, no attention was paid by the military to venereal disease. It was during World War I that the U.S. War Department first sought to protect soldiers from venereal disease, then the symbol of social decadence. The movement against venereal disease became the most eloquent endeavor in social engineering in the history of the United States. Proper moral behavior and magic bullets, polar opposites, were embraced in the name of the family.

Between 1880 and 1980, nonsexually-transmitted diseases such as diphtheria, dysentery, pneumonia, tuberculosis, and typhoid were conquered. Brandt wonders why nonsexually-transmitted infectious diseases have been defeated and venereal diseases such as AIDS, gonorrhea, herpes, and syphilis continue to spread. The battle against venereal disease is complicated by factors associated with class, culture, economics, ethnicity, gender, politics, and race which far outweigh the strength of magic bullets.

The history of syphilis in the early 1900s seems relevant to the current consideration of AIDS. AIDS has no available cure and results in death. Education and social engineering are the only available means to impede the epidemic. Because there is no magic bullet, dismay, dread, and fear abound, magnifying ingrained cultural and social apprehension.

Brandt has placed AIDS within a historical context. One can admire his unique contribution and clearly stated thesis.

SOCIOLOGY

Dennis Altman, a political scientist and author of books on the Gay community, has written *AIDS in the Mind of America: The Social, Political, and Psychological Impact of a New Epidemic*. He contends that disease has important political ramifications. For example, heart transplants for middle- and upper-class citizens, paid for by third-party insurance payments, are seen as a more acceptable allocation of funds than the sickle-cell anemia or lead poisoning common among noninsured lower-class persons.

During this century, the civil rights obtained in local and state governments for gays and lesbians occurred because gay white men, knowledgeable about working within the system, were able to provide their expertise to the movement. In 1969, the Stonewall riots in New York City influenced gays and lesbians to come out of the closet with a new sense of pride and power. However, just as being gay was becoming less of a stigma, AIDS emerged. At first, from October 1980 to September 1982, AIDS was called GRIDS (Gay-Related Immunodeficiency Syndrome) by the Centers for Disease Control. It took 2 years for the name AIDS (Acquired Immunodeficiency Syndrome) to reflect the nonexclusivity of the disease.

Because, unlike drug users, Haitians, and hemophiliacs, gay men had the visible community organization, resources, and political knowledge with which to respond to the AIDS crisis, AIDS became associated with the Gay community. Previously nonpolitical individuals became political and skilled leaders emerged. However, gays lacked the mass appeal necessary to achieve crucial governmental involvement. President Reagan telephoned Rock Hudson before he died, but continued to see AIDS as a gay problem rather than as a public health crisis. Gay groups have done more to provide counseling, education, home health care, and hot lines to gay and nongay AIDS clients than have the country's public health agencies.

Altman sees AIDS as the first of many new syndromes which directly stem from the technological age. Some researchers believe that years of ingestion of antibiotics, actively through medical administration and passively through food intake, have lowered the immune system's ability to work properly.

AIDS is teaching governments how to respond to a medical emergency. However, despite the urgent pleas from gay groups, the National Institutes of Health did not call for AIDS research proposals until August 1982, and did not begin funding until 1983. The Food and Drug Administration did not license tests for antibodies to HIV until Spring 1985.

The manner in which society deals with AIDS will mirror its attitudes. For instance, in mid-1800 Great Britain, the Contagious Diseases Acts demanded that "licentious women" be examined and registered every 2 weeks. In 1900 San Francisco, the plague led to the quarantine of Chinatown. Today, HIV antibody test results could be used to quarantine individuals who test positive and to deny them employment, insurance, and marriage licenses.

AIDS in the Mind of America is one of the first books to describe the sociological aspects of AIDS. In it, Altman presents a rational history of AIDS, indicating how society's reactions are more a reflection of its values than of unbiased medical facts. AIDS presents a challenge not just to the individuals it attacks but to human civilization itself.

POLITICS

A casual browser at the library might look at the 630-page book, *And the Band Played On: Politics, People, and the AIDS Epidemic*, and bypass it for a thinner volume on the subject of AIDS. This would be a mistake.

Randy Shilts was a reporter for the *San Francisco Chronicle*, one of the first daily newspapers not to require the death of a movie star to make AIDS a valid news story. In *And the Band Played On*, Shilts reports the history of AIDS from July 4, 1976, to May 31, 1987. A thorough journalist, Shilts clothes his text with a description of the bureaucracy and the dramatis personae, 900 interviewees, meterological details, sources, and an index. A creative dramatist, he dresses the document with anecdotes, dialogue, gossip, parables, quotations, and stories.

On October 2, 1985, Rock Hudson died. A few months before his death, when the diagnosis of his illness was announced to the world, the mainstream press finally acknowledged the presence of the AIDS epidemic. By that time, 12,000 Americans had died from or been diagnosed with AIDS. By the time President Reagan finally gave his first speech on AIDS on May 31, 1987, 36,058 Americans had been diagnosed with AIDS and 20,849 had died.

Shilts details the many failures and few successes in the early years of research on AIDS, particularly noteworthy given the availability of the world's most refined medical resources and most developed public health system. Local public health authorities thought of AIDS as a political issue. Gay leaders determined AIDS to be a public relations problem. The media hesitated to devote space to stories on gay life, especially gay sexual practices, and assumed that AIDS would not be of interest to the general public. Chaos ensued, due more to ineptitude than to any particular maliciousness toward the individuals with AIDS.

Two stars emerge in the story: Dr. C. Everett Koop and Dr. Mathilde Krim. In 1986, Dr. Koop, a religious conservative and supporter of the anti-abortion movement, devoted much of his time to interviewing medical professionals on AIDS. He then wrote and published, without White House clearance, the *Surgeon General's Report on Acquired Immune Deficiency Syndrome* (Koop, 1986) in which he recommended condoms, confidential testing, and AIDS education. Dr. Krim, the researcher known as the "interferon queen" at the Memorial Sloan-Kettering Cancer Center, was appalled at the inadequacy of response and coordination of services in New York City. Married to Arthur Krim, Chairman of the Board for Orion Pictures, she had the social connections which would help her raise sufficient funds to establish the American Foundation for AIDS Research and to promote effective care of individuals with AIDS.

And the Band Played On should be viewed as basic required reading on AIDS. I found it difficult to put down and, when I finished it, I wanted to read more. A few months after reading it, I find more retention of information from this book than from any other on AIDS that I have read. I look forward to reading Randy Shilts' future melodies.

MEDIA

James Baldwin, in his 1978 book *The Devil Finds Work*, wrote that "the victim who is able to articulate the situation of the victim has ceased to be a victim; he, or she, has become a threat." In *Policing Desire: Pornography, AIDS, and the Media*, Simon Watney, Professor of Communication History and Theory of Photography, analyzes the role of the press in the accounting of AIDS in Great Britain and the United States. The war against AIDS is not limited to medical diagnosis and treatment. "It involves our understanding of the words and images which load the virus down with such a dismal cargo of appalling connotations." Watney describes the images used by the press to refer to AIDS, noting that the symbols used when discussing AIDS have a powerful impact on public reaction. His requests to newspapers for permission to reprint cartoons and photographs in the book were either ignored or rejected.

Historically, Great Britain has persecuted groups it hosted who were not like its middle and upper classes: Blacks, Christian sectarians, gays, gypsies, Jews, the mad, prostitutes, and witches. Each persecuted group has been described as erotic, indecent, depraved, and unclean. The Human Immunodeficiency Virus initially revealed itself in three minorities who already were denigrated and mistrusted as peripheral members of society—Blacks, recreational drug users, and gay men.

Persons with AIDS are divided into two distinct categories by the press: (a) the innocent "victims," e.g., hemophiliacs, children, and unknowing heterosexual partners of drug users and ambisexuals, and (b) the guilty spreaders, e.g., homosexual men and recreational IV drug users. Hospital policies are developed more to protect the "innocent" staff than the "guilty" AIDS patient.

Watney suggests that the terms "smart sex" and "safer sex" are more accurate than "safe sex." He recommends that safer sex be promoted by associating it with symbols connoting comfort, nurturance, and passion. The incorporation of condoms in seductive advertisements, television, porno shows, posters, telephone sex, and theatrical presentations could foster the inclusion of condoms in private reverie.

Watney provides an in-depth analysis of AIDS within the context of current American and British views on sexuality. He presents good information, but in a somewhat long-winded manner.

MEDICAL SCIENCE

AIDS was the theme of the October, 1985, annual meeting of the Institute of Medicine. During that meeting, it was recognized that under the Congressional charter which established the National Academy of Science, it could develop recommendations regarding research directions for AIDS and the care of persons with AIDS. The papers of the meeting itself have been edited into a nontechnical volume entitled, *Mobilizing Against AIDS: The Unfinished Story of a Virus*. The recommendations constructed after the meeting have been edited into the volume, *Confronting AIDS: Directions for Public Health, Health Care, and Research*. The second volume contains information of a broader scope than the first, is clear and readable, and, for individuals wishing to choose between the two, is preferred.

In *Confronting AIDS*, the following areas are discussed: the status, dimensions, and future course of the epidemic; opportunities for affecting the future course; required research; international developments; and care of the AIDS client. The two major recommendations are that:

1. The U.S. federal government spend $1 billion a year on an education, media, and public health campaign to prevent the further spread of AIDS.
2. The U.S. federal government spend $1 billion a year on long-term biological, medical, and social science research designed to prevent and to treat AIDS.

Confronting AIDS is an excellent condensation of the state of scientific thought about AIDS as of 1986. A new volume, *Confronting AIDS: Update 1988*, was released in June 1988.

NUTRITION

Scientific nutritional assessment and treatment of AIDS is abridged into a timesaver publication for health professionals published by Ross Laboratories called *Dietetic Currents*. Candy L. Collins presents in five pages a summary article of her work and research as a registered dietitian with AIDS clients. Most valuable is the list of over forty medical references for specialized reading.

HOSPICE CARE

Elisabeth Kübler-Ross, a psychiatrist who has written extensively on death and dying, has written *AIDS: The Ultimate Challenge*. Kübler-Ross indicates that her work with AIDS clients is different from her work with others. Persons with AIDS generally have a shorter prognosis and go through the stages of death and dying to inner peace more quickly than clients with a longer prognosis. "What this epidemic teaches us is to become honest again, to talk and listen to each other, to accept and love each other more and, most important, to learn to get our priorities straight."

Kübler-Ross writes of her work with gays and notes that, with her clientele, one-half of the mothers and one-third of the fathers, upon hearing that their son was gay and had AIDS, accepted and supported them. AIDS presents families with an opportunity to learn to express amity, understanding, love, mercy, and sympathy. Persons with AIDS must learn to accept that they are ill, to love themselves, and to allow themselves the freedom to do what they need to do for their own well-being.

In her book, Kübler-Ross devotes chapters specifically to babies, children, women, and prisoners with AIDS. Much of the book is related to her attempt and failure to organize a hospice for abandoned babies with AIDS at her home in Head Waters, Virginia. She had wished to create a place for them to live in love and nature for their short lives rather than spend their entire lives isolated in hospital cribs. She describes the pressure from hospital administrators who preferred to make financial profits on the care of the baby rather than to allow the child to be placed with an adoptive family. She experienced the fear in her home community of associating with HIV-infected persons. A transcript of the public hearing and letters to the local newspaper fill the book. This book may be helpful for individuals who live in middle America and who have not yet read much about AIDS.

Kübler-Ross' emphasis is on the dying process. There are many, however, who would like more acknowledgement of the fact that a number of persons with AIDS have not died. In 1985, physician and cautious writer, Jean Shinoda Bolen, traced the healing process of one individual who had had a diagnosis of AIDS. In 1988, Oprah Winfrey devoted one of her television shows to "AIDS and Self Healing," interviewing several persons with AIDS who had reversed the course of the disease. In essence, these individuals have created a self-affirmative field, emphasizing quality of life and employing such tools as imagery, relaxation, physical exercise, nutrition, and play (Hay, 1988; Jeter, 1981; Levine, 1987). A support system which challenges, informs, and nurtures is particularly important. *The People With AIDS Coalition Newsline* lists support groups, holistic support, recreational activities, treatment centers, and ministries as well as provides a forum for the sharing of experience and thought.

YOUTH EDUCATION

Oralee Wachter, producer of films for youth on such issues as acquaintance rape, adolescent pregnancy, and sexual abuse, has produced a film and written a book, both entitled, *Sex, Drugs, and AIDS*. She bases her work on the October, 1986, *Surgeon General's Report on AIDS* (Koop, 1986). The book and film are narrated by Rae Dawn Chong and have been praised by Phil Donahue, C. Everett Koop, Mathilde Krim, Abigail Van Buren, and others. The message is "AIDS is hard to get." You have to "put" the virus in your blood through drugs or sex. Emphasis is on heterosexual sex and teenage girls are depicted having a conversation about "the first time." Five risk groups are indicated—gays and ambisexuals, intravenous drug users, people who have received infected blood transfusions, sexual partners of individuals in high-risk groups, and babies born to infected mothers. As it states, "Well, there's nobody to blame except the virus."

The film, *Sex, Drugs, and AIDS*, is an excellent way to introduce the topic of AIDS to youth. As the rates for gonorrhea and syphilis increase in the urban barrios and ghettos, it is clear that our sex education needs significant reevaluation and redirection. Audio-visuals such as this film will be appropriate instructional media.

ADULT EDUCATION

John Preston, Past Managing Editor of *SIECUS Report* and graduate of the University of Minnesota Medical School Human Sexuality Program, collaborates with "Mr. Safe Sex," Glenn Swann, to author, *Safe Sex: The Ultimate Erotic Guide*, one of the more amusing and blunt "how-to" books on the market. With the concern about possible anonymous sex in bath houses, the Club Baths Chain was renamed the Club Body Centers and emphasis was placed on body building, community endeavors, and educational programs.

Former U.S. Marine and pornography star, Glenn Swann, was selected to be Mr. Safe Sex.

Preston and Swann agree that defining sex as sexual intercourse is like playing only one type of music; there are options. So, for instance, if disco music were to be proclaimed dangerous, other forms of music such as blues, country, jazz, opera, ragtime, rock-and-roll, and spirituals would be available.

The book follows Mr. Safe Sex on his national tour, learning and teaching, discovering and employing such alternatives as condoms, dildos, fantasy, heterosexuality, massage, monogamy, mutual masturbation, romance, stimulation of nipples, stripping, telephone sex, vibrators, and wrestling. Wearing his Marine issue boots, jacket, and jock strap, he appears before audiences who probably are not reading literature or listening to lectures on safe sex. Sergeant Swann bellows out in the best Lejeune tradition, "You can't do those things any more. We have buddies who are in trouble, and we have to help them! We have to learn how to take care of ourselves, and we have to learn how to be careful of others as well. Stop doing the things that make you and our buddies sick!"

The rules are indisputable:

1. Do not swallow semen.
2. Use condoms.
3. Do not consume urine.
4. Do not play with your confidante's sex toys.
5. Do not have oral-anal contact ("rim").

This book is a fun safe-sex come-on. The photographs by Fred Bissones are true pin-ups. This is not a book of intellectual depth, nor is it meant to be. Rather, it wraps the safe sex message in a jock strap for light pornographic reading.

The Gay Men's Health Crisis Center also has employed light pornography to educate individuals about safer sex in a video called *Chance of a Lifetime*. Viewers learn to have fun with condoms during sex play. The audience is asked to place condoms on all the penises in their fantasy and real-life interludes.

CONCLUSION

The resources on AIDS mentioned in this review contain vast amounts of information about the epidemiology, virology, treatment, history, sociology and psychology of AIDS. Meanwhile, men and women from all over the world carefully embroider their experience of AIDS and stitch it into the National Names Project/ AIDS Quilt which is housed in San Francisco and now on traveling exhibit. Their careful piecing together of truth recalls, for me, the Egyptian myth of Isis, found in the Pyramid Texts which originated in the third millennium B.C.E. and were inscribed in stone around 2300 B.C.E. (see Houston, in press; Stone, 1976).

In the beginning there was Isis, Oldest of the Old. She was the Goddess from whom all becoming arose. Isis, the Mother Goddess, the Thousand-Named, created all the objects which lightened the human's toil on earth. While Isis governed Egypt, her brother and husband, Osiris, taught the Egyptians how to use Isis' tools.

Their jealous brother, Seth, nailed Osiris into a wooden coffin and then cut him into fourteen pieces, scattering them around the Mediterranean Sea. Isis wept, causing the Nile to flow over the desert. She surveyed the known world, locating one piece after another. Carefully, Isis reassembled Osiris, except for his lost penis. Isis created and fired a penis of clay and presented Osiris with this new life power. She then inseminated herself and bore their son, Horus.

Thus, life continues, generation after generation, even unto today, due to Isis' caring. Each June as the Nile floods, the Night of the Tear-Drop is celebrated, commemorating Isis' genuine concern for Osiris and the vital life force of the universe.

The ancient archetype of Isis stands as a role model for our response to AIDS. The crisis requires that we weep for the lost lives, diligently search for and piece together the truth, and reconnect with the universal life force. AIDS presents us with the ultimate challenge.

REFERENCES

"AIDS and self healing" [*Oprah Winfrey Show*]. (1988, Spring). Chicago, IL: WLS-TV.

Altman, D. (1986). *AIDS in the mind of America: The social, political, and psychological impact of a new epidemic.* Garden City, NY: Anchor Press/Doubleday.

Baldwin, J. (1976). *The devil finds work.* New York: Dial Press.

Black, D. (1985). *The plague years: A chronicle of AIDS, the epidemic of our times.* New York: Simon and Schuster.

Bolen, J. S. (1985, March/April). William Calderon: Incredible triumph over AIDS brings new hope. *New Realities,* pp. 8-15.

Brandt, A. M. (1987). *No magic bullet: A social history of venereal disease in the United States since 1880 with a new chapter on AIDS.* Expanded Edition. New York: Oxford University Press.

Chance of a lifetime. (1985). New York: Gay Men's Health Crisis Center.

Collins, C. (1988). Nutrition care in AIDS. *Dietetic Currents, 15,* 3.

Hay, L. L. (1988). *The AIDS book: Creating a positive approach.* Santa Monica, CA: Hay House.

Houston, Jean (in press). *Isis and Osiris: The passion play of ancient egypt.* Warwick, NY: Amity House.

Institute of Medicine, National Academy of Sciences. (1986). *Confronting AIDS: Directions for public health, health care, and research.* Washington, DC: National Academy Press.

Institute of Medicine, National Academy of Sciences. (1988). *Confronting AIDS: Update 1988.* Washington, DC: National Academy Press.

Jeter, K. (1981). Family medicine and holistic health. In B. E. Cogswell & M. B. Sussman (Eds.), *Family medicine: A new approach to health care.* New York: The Haworth Press.

Koop, C. E. (1986). *Surgeon General's Report on Acquired Immune Deficiency Syndrome.* Washington, DC: U.S. Public Health Service.

Kübler-Ross, E. (1987). *AIDS: The ultimate challenge.* New York: Macmillan.

Levine, S. (1987). *Healing into life and death.* New York: Doubleday.

Nichols, E. K. (1986). *Mobilizing against AIDS: The unfinished story of a virus.* Cambridge, MA: Harvard University Press.

People With AIDS Coalition Newsline. (1986, ongoing). New York: Gay and Lesbian Press Association.

Preston, J., & Swann, G. (1986). *Safe Sex: The ultimate erotic guide.* New York: New American Library.

Shilts, R. (1987). *And the band played on: Politics, people, and the AIDS epidemic.* New York: St. Martin's Press.

Stone, M. (1976). *When God was a woman.* New York: Dial Press.

Wachter, O. (1987). *Sex, drugs, and AIDS.* New York: Bantam Books.

Watney, S. (1987). *Policing desire: Pornography, AIDS, and the media.* Minneapolis, MN: University of Minnesota Press.

Listing of Resources

BOOKS

Altman, D. (1986). *AIDS in the mind of America*. Garden City, NY: Doubleday.

Alyson, S. (Ed.) (1988). *You can do something about AIDS*. Boston: Alyson Publications.

American Psychologist. (1988, November), *43*. (Special issue: Psychology and AIDS.)

Bridge, T. P., Mirsky, A. F., & Goodwin, F. K. (Eds.) (1988). *Psychological, neuropsychiatric, and substance abuse aspects of AIDS*. New York: Raven Press.

Buckingham, S. (Ed.) (1988). AIDS: A special issue of *Social Casework*, *69*(6), 324-408.

Callen, M. (Ed.) (1987). *Surviving and thriving with AIDS: Hints for the newly diagnosed*. New York: People With AIDS Coalition, Inc.

Dalton, H. L., & Burris, S. (Eds.) (1987). *AIDS and the law*. New Haven, CT: Yale University Press.

Delaney, M., & Goldblum, P. (1987). *Strategies for survival: A gay men's health manual for the age of AIDS*. New York: St. Martin's Press.

Eidson, T. (Ed.) (1988). *The AIDS caregiver's handbook*. New York: St. Martin's Press.

Galea, R. P., Lewis, B. F., & Baker, L. A. (Eds.) (1987). *AIDS and IV drug abusers: Current perspectives*. Owings Mills, MD: Rynd Communications.

Griggs, J. (Ed.) (1986). *AIDS: Public policy dimensions*. Based on Proceedings of the National Conference Sponsored by the United Hospital Fund and the Institute for Health Policy Studies, N.Y.C. (Write: Publications Program, United Hospital Fund of New York, 55 Fifth Ave., New York, NY 10003.)

Hay, L. L. (1988). *The AIDS book: Creating a positive approach.* Santa Monica, CA: Hay House.

Helmquist, M. (1987). *Working with AIDS: A resource guide for mental health professionals.* San Francisco, CA: AIDS Project, University of California.

Institute of Medicine, National Academy of Sciences. (1986). *Confronting AIDS: Directions for public health, health care, and research.* Washington, DC: National Academy Press. (Write: 2101 Constitution Ave., N.W., Washington, DC 20418.)

Institute of Medicine, National Academy of Sciences. (1988). *Confronting AIDS: Update 1988.* Washington, DC: National Academy Press.

Kelly, J. A., & St. Lawrence, J. (1988). *The AIDS health crisis: Psychological and social intervention.* New York: Plenum.

Martelli, L. J., Peltz, F. D. P., & Messina, W. (1987). *When someone you know has AIDS.* New York: Crown Publishers.

McKusick, L. (Ed.) (1986). *What to do about AIDS: Physicians and mental health professionals discuss the issues.* Berkeley, CA: University of California Press.

Moffatt, B. C. (1986). *When someone you love has AIDS: A book of hope for family and friends.* New York: NAL Penguin, Inc.

Moffatt, B. C. (Ed.) (1987). *AIDS: A self-care manual.* Santa Monica, CA: IBS Press.

New England Journal of Public Policy. (1988, Winter/Spring), *4*(1), 525 pp. (Special issue on AIDS.)

Nichols, E. K. (1986). *Mobilizing against AIDS: The unfinished story of a virus.* Cambridge, MA: Harvard University Press.

Norwood, C. (1987). *Advice for life: A woman's guide to AIDS risks and prevention.* New York: Pantheon Books.

Patton, C. (1986). *Sex and germs: The politics of AIDS.* Boston: South End Press.

Peabody, B. (1986). *The screaming room: Mother's journal of her son's struggle with AIDS.* San Diego: Oak Tree Publications (New York: Avon Books, 1987).

Pierce, C., & Van de Veer, D. (1987). *AIDS: Ethics and public policy.* Belmont, CA: Wadsworth Publishing Company.

Science. (1988, February 5), *239*, 533-696. (Special issue on AIDS.)

Scientific American. (1988, October), *259*, 152pp. (Special issue on AIDS.)

Shilts, R. (1987). *And the band played on.* New York: St. Martin's Press.

Watkins, J. D. et al. (1988). *Report of the Presidential Commission on the Human Immunodeficiency Virus Epidemic.* (Write: Presidential Commission, 655 15th Street N.W., Suite 901, Washington, DC 20005.)

Whitmore, G. (1988). *Someone was here: Profiles in the AIDs epidemic.* New York: NAL Books/New American Library.

Witt, M. D. (Ed.) (1986). *AIDS and patient management: Legal, ethical, and social issues.* Owings Mills, MD: National Health Publications.

PAMPHLETS FOR FAMILIES AND CAREGIVERS

AIDS and Children: Information for Parents of School-age Children. (1986). American Red Cross, AIDS Public Education Program, 1730 E Street N.W., Washington, DC 20006. (202) 639-3223. 5 pp.

AIDS: Helping Families Cope. (1988). National Association of Social Workers, 7981 Eastern Avenue, Silver Springs, MD 20910. (301) 565-0333. 10pp. (plus videotape).

Caring for the AIDS Patient at Home. (1986). American Red Cross, AIDS Public Education Program, 1730 E Street N.W., Washington, DC 20006. (202) 639-3223. 6 pp.

Children With AIDS: Guidelines for Parents and Caregivers. (1986). The AIDS Task Force of Central New York, P.O. Box 1911, Syracuse, NY 13201. 12 pp.

Coping with AIDS: Psychological and Social Considerations in Helping People with HTLV III Infection. (1986). National Institute of Mental Health, Office of Scientific Information, 5600 Fisher's Lane, Rockville, MD 20857. 19 pp.

How to Talk to Your Children About AIDS. (1986). SIECUS, 32 Washington Place, Room 52, New York, NY 10003. (212) 673-3850. 6 pp.

I Can't Cope With My Fear of AIDS. (1986). Gay Men's Health

Crisis, Inc., Box 274, 132 West 24th Street, New York, NY 10011. (212) 807-6655. 4 pp.

Lesbians and AIDS: What's the Connection? (1986). San Francisco AIDS Foundation, 333 Valencia Street, 4th Flr., San Francisco, CA 94103. (415) 864-6606. 4 pp.

No-Nonsense AIDS Answers. (1987). Written by Robert W. Windom and C. Everett Koop for Blue Cross/Blue Shield Association, 676 North St. Clair Street, Chicago, IL 60611. 11 pp.

Sourcebook on Lesbian/Gay Health Care. National Lesbian/Gay Health Foundation, P.O. Box 65472, Washington, DC 20035. ($15.00, prepaid.)

Surgeon General's Report on Acquired Immune Deficiency Syndrome. (1986). U.S. Public Health Service, Public Affairs Office, Hubert H. Humphrey Blvd., Room 725H, 200 Independence Avenue S.W., Washington, DC 20201. (202) 245-6867. 36 pp.

The Facilitator's Guide to Eroticizing Safer Sex: A Psychoeducational Workshop Model. Gay Men's Health Crisis, Inc., Box 274, 132 West 24th Street, New York, NY 10011. (212) 807-6655. ($8.00, prepaid.)

Understanding AIDS: A Message From the Surgeon General, (1988). U.S. Department of Health and Human Services, Public Health Service, Centers for Disease Control, P. O. Box 6003, Rockville, MD 20850. 8 pp.

What Parents Need To Tell Children About AIDS. (1987). The AIDS Institute, New York State Health Department, Empire State Plaza, Corning Tower, Room 359, Albany, NY 12237. (518) 474-3045. 12 pp.

When A Friend Has AIDS. (1986). Gay Men's Health Crisis, Inc., Box 274, 132 West 24th Street, New York, NY 10011. (212) 807-6655. 4 pp.

When A Friend Has AIDS. American Association for Counseling and Development, 5999 Stevenson Ave., Alexandria, VA 22304. (800) 354-2008. 4 pp.

Women and AIDS. (1987). The AIDS Institute, New York State Health Department, Empire State Plaza, Corning Tower, Room 359, Albany, NY 12237. (518) 474-3045. 2 pp.

Women Need to Know About AIDS. (1986). Gay Men's Health Crisis, Inc., Box 274, 132 West 24th Street, New York, NY 10011. (212) 807-6655. 4 pp.

What You Should Know About AIDS: Facts About the Disease, How to Protect Yourself and Your Family, What To Tell Others. (1987). America Responds to AIDS, P. O. Box 6003, Rockville, MD 20850. (800) 342-7514. 7 pp.

Your Child and AIDS. (1986). San Francisco AIDS Foundation, 333 Valencia Street, 4th Floor, San Francisco, CA 94103. (415) 864-4376. 6 pp.

NEWSLETTERS AND PERIODICALS

AAPHR Letter, American Association of Physicians for Human Rights, P.O. Box 14366, San Francisco, CA 94114. (415) 558-9353. ($125, Quarterly).

AIDS: An International Bimonthly Journal, Grower Academic Journals, 34 Cleveland Street, LONDON, W1P 5FB, United Kingdom. ($30, Bimonthly).

AIDS & ARC News, Belmont Publishing Co., 1059 Alameda, Belmont, CA 94002. (415) 591-0935. ($95, Monthly).

AIDS and Public Policy Journal, University Publishing Group, 107 E. Church Street, Frederick, MD 21701. (800) 654-8188. ($95, Quarterly).

AIDS Education and Prevention: An Interdisciplinary Journal, Guilford Publications, Inc., 72 Spring Street, New York, NY 10012. (800) 221-3966.

AIDS Law and Litigation Reporter, University Publishing Group, 107 E. Church Street, Frederick, MD 21701. (800) 654-8188. ($450).

AIDS Literature and News Review, University Publishing Group, 107 E. Church Street, Frederick, MD 21701. (800) 654-8188. ($185).

AIDS Patient Care, Mary Ann Liebert, Inc., 1651 Third Ave., New York, NY 10128. (212) 289-2300. ($90, Bimonthly).

AIDS Policy and Law, Buraff Publications, Inc., 2445 M Street NW, Washington, DC 20037. (202) 728-3360. ($387, Bimonthly).

AIDS Record, Bio-Data Publishers, 1518 K Street NW, Washington, DC 20005. (202) 783-0110. ($275, Biweekly).

AIDS Reference and Research Collection, University Publishing Group, 107 E. Church Street, Frederick, MD 21701. (800) 654-8188. ($185).

AIDS Reference Guide: A Sourcebook for Planners and Decision Makers, Atlanta Information Services, Inc., 1050 17th Street, N.W., Suite 480, Washington, DC 20036. (800) 521-4323. ($389, Monthly).

AIDS Targeted Information Newsletter, Williams and Wilkins, P.O. Box 23291, Baltimore, MD 21203. (800) 638-6423. ($125, Monthly).

AIDS Update, Lambda Legal Defense and Education Fund, Inc., 132 W. 43rd Street, New York, NY 10036. (212) 944-9488. ($50, Monthly).

CDC AIDS Weekly, P.O. Box 5528, Atlanta, GA 30307-0528. ($520, Weekly).

Children with AIDS Newsletter, Foundation for Children with AIDS, Inc., 77B Warren Street, Brighton, MA 02135. (617) 783-7300. ($15, Quarterly).

Focus: A Guide to AIDS Research, FOCUS Subscriptions, UCSF AIDS Health Project, Box 0884, San Francisco, CA 94143-0884. ($36, monthly).

Journal of Acquired Immune Deficiency Syndromes, Raven Press, Dept. 1B, 1185 Avenue of the Americas, New York, NY 10109-0012. ($85, Bimonthly).

NAPWA News, National Association of People with AIDS, 1012 14th Street NW, Suite 601, Washington, DC 20005. ($25, Quarterly).

Network News, National AIDS Network, 1012 14th Street NW, Washington, DC 20005. (202) 347-0390. ($100, Semi-monthly).

AUDIO-VISUAL MATERIALS

1. *AIDS: A Family Experience*. (1988). Videotape—35 minutes. Rental $75; purchase price $395. Distributor: Carle Medical Communications, 110 W. Main Street, Urbana, IL 61801. (217)

384-4838. How one family coped with having a member with AIDS.

2. *AIDS: Changing the Rules*. (1987). Videotape — 28 minutes or 60 minutes. Purchase price $30 or $45. Teacher guide available. Distributor: WETA Educational Activities, P. O. Box 2626, Washington, DC 20013. (800) 445-1964. Documentary about the risk and prevention of AIDS in heterosexual adults, starring Ron Reagan, Jr., Beverly Johnson, and Ruben Blades.

3. *AIDS: Our Fears, Our Hopes*. Script available from: Family Service America, 11700 W. Lake Park Drive, Milwaukee, WI 53224. (414) 359-2111. A drama written by Family Service of Philadelphia, Plays for Living Division.

4. *The AIDS Movie*. (1986). 16mm film or videotape — 26 minutes. Rental $57; purchase price $385. Distributor: New Day Films, 2 Riverview Drive, Wayne, NJ 07470. (201) 633-0212. Interviews with three persons with AIDS.

5. *AIDS: What Everyone Needs to Know* (Revised). (1987). 16mm film or videotape — 20 minutes. Rental $60; purchase price for film $395; for videotape $275. For purchase: Churchill Films, 662 North Robertson Blvd., Los Angeles, CA 90069. (213) 657-5110 (in CA), (800) 334-7830 (outside CA). For rental: Audience Planners, 5107 Douglas Fir Road, Calabasas, CA 91302. (818) 884-3100 (in CA), (800) 624-8613 (outside CA).

6. *A Letter From Brian*. (1987). Videotape — 30 minutes. Rental $8; purchase price $95. Contact your local Red Cross chapter or the national office in Washington, DC (see National Resources). For high school and college students.

7. *An Ounce of Prevention: How To Talk With A Partner About Smart Sex*. (1988). Audiotape by Bernie Zilbergeld and Lonnie Barbach. Distributor: Fay Institute, 80 Ogden Avenue, Dobbs Ferry, NY 10522. (800) 341-1950 (ext. 88). Vignettes of possible conversations with sexual partners about safer-sex techniques.

8. *Male Couples Facing AIDS*. (1988). Videotape — 30 minutes. Developed by Andrew M. Mattison and David P. McWhirter. Distributor: Mariposa Education & Research Foundation, 4545 Park Blvd., Suite 207, San Diego, CA 92116. (619) 542-0088. Documentary about male couples in which one or both partners has AIDS. (Also includes Discussion Guide.)

9. *Sex, Drugs, and AIDS*. (1986). 16mm film or videotape — 18 minutes. Rental $75; purchase price $325 for tape; $400 for film. Distributor: ODN Productions, 74 Varick Street, Suite 304, New York, NY 10013. (212) 431-8923.

10. *Too Little, Too Late*. (1987). Videotape — 48 minutes. Rental $75; purchase price $400. Distributor: Fanlight Productions, 47 Halifax Street, Boston, MA 02130. (617) 524-0980. Documentary about families of persons with AIDS.

ORGANIZATIONS

1. AIDS Action Institute, 729 8th Street SE, Suite 200, Washington, DC 20003. (202) 547-3101.

2. AIDS and Civil Liberties Project, Civil Liberties Union, 132 West 43rd Street, New York, NY 10036. (212) 944-9800.

3. AIDS Hotline for Kids, Center for Attitudinal Healing, 19 Main Street, Tiburon, CA 94920. (415) 435-5022.

4. AIDS Information Resources Directory. Available free from: AmFAR, Suite 406, 40 W. 57th Street, New York, NY 10019. (212) 333-3118.

5. The AIDS Institute, New York State Health Department, Empire State Plaza, Corning Tower, Room 359, Albany, NY 12237. (518) 473-7238 (general); (518) 474-3045 (education materials). Clearinghouse for materials published by New York State.

6. AIDS Project, Ackerman Institute for Family Therapy, 149 East 78th Street, New York, NY 10021. (212) 879-4900.

7. America Responds to AIDS, P. O. Box 6003, Rockville, MD 20850. (800) 342-7514.

8. American College Health Association, 15879 Crabbs Branch Way, Rockville, MD 20855. (301) 963-1100.

9. American Foundation for AIDS Research (AmFAR), 40 W. 57th Street, Suite 406, New York, NY 10019. (212) 333-3118.

10. American Red Cross, AIDS Public Education Program, 1730 E Street N.W., Washington, DC 20006. (202) 639-3223.

11. Association of Drug Abuse Prevention and Treatment (ADAPT), 85 Bergen Street, Brooklyn, NY 11201. (718) 834-9585.

12. Centers for Disease Control (AIDS Program), 1600 Clifton

Road NE, Atlanta, GA 30333. (404) 639-2891 (general information); (404) 639-1388 (photographic slides); (404) 639-3534 (public inquiries); (404) 639-3472 (*AIDS Weekly Surveillance Report*).

13. Computer AIDS Information Network (CAIN), 1213 North Highland Avenue, Hollywood, CA 90038. (213) 464-7400. For subscription, write to: General Videotex, 3 Blackstone Street, Cambridge, MA 02139. (800) 544-4005.

14. Foundation for Children With AIDS, Inc., 77B Warren Street, Brighton, MA 02135. (617) 783-7300.

15. Gay Men's Health Crisis (GMHC), Box 274, 132 West 24th Street, New York, NY 10011. (212) 807-6655/7517.

16. HERO (Health Education Resource Organization), 100 Maryland Avenue, Suite 240, Rockville, MD 20850. (301) 762-3385.

17. Lambda Legal Defense and Education Fund, 666 Broadway, 12th Floor, New York, NY 10012. (212) 995-8585.

18. Minority Task Force on AIDS, 92 St. Nichols Ave., Apt. 1B, New York, NY 10026. (212) 749-2816.

19. Mothers of AIDS Patients (MAP), c/o Barbara Peabody, 3403 E Street, San Diego, CA 92102. (619) 293-3985.

20. National AIDS Hotline (sponsored by Federal Centers for Disease Control/American Social Health Association), (800) 342-AIDS for general AIDS-related information: (800) 342-7514 for AIDS information and referral services for counseling and testing.

21. National AIDS Information Clearinghouse, U.S. Public Health Service, Rockville, MD (301) 762-5111.

22. National AIDS Network, 1012 14th Street NW, Suite 601, Washington, DC 20005. (202) 347-0390.

23. National Association of People with AIDS, 2025 I Street NW, Suite 415, Washington, DC 20006. (202) 429-2856, (202) 347-1317.

24. National Coalition on AIDS and Families, c/o Marriage and Family Therapy Program, 008 Slocum Hall, Syracuse University, Syracuse, NY 13244-1250. (315) 443-3023.

25. National Council of Churches AIDS Task Force, 475 Riverside Drive, Room 572, New York, NY 10115. (212) 870-2385.

26. National Hemophilia Foundation, 110 Greene Street, Room 406, New York, NY 10012. (212) 219-8180.

27. National Leadership Coalition on AIDS, 1150 17th Street N.W., Suite 202, Washington, DC 20036. (202) 429-0930.

28. National Lesbian and Gay Health Foundation, P. O. Box 65472, Washington, DC 20035. (202) 797-3708.

29. Parents and Friends of Lesbians and Gays (PFLAG), c/o Paulette Goodman, P. O. Box 3533, Silver Springs, MD 20901. (301) 439-3524.

30. People With AIDS Coalition, Inc., 263A West 19th Street, Room 125, New York, NY 10011. (212) 627-1810.

31. San Francisco AIDS Foundation, 333 Valencia Street, 4th Floor, San Francisco, CA 94103. (415) 864-4376.

32. Shanti Project, 525 Howard Street, San Francisco, CA 94105-3080. (415) 777-2273.

33. SIECUS (Sex Information & Education Council of the U.S.), 32 Washington Place, New York, NY 10003. (212) 673-3850.

34. U.S. Public Health Service, 200 Independence Avenue SW, Washington, DC 20201. (202) 245-6867 — Office of Communications, Room 725H (press office for Assistant Secretary of Health and the Surgeon General); (202) 245-0471 — AIDS Coordinator, Room 729H.

35. Visiting Nurses and Hospice of San Francisco, Fox Plaza, 1390 Market Street, Suite 510, San Francisco, CA 94102. (415) 861-8705. (Publishes AIDS Home-care and Hospice Manual.)

Members of the AIDS Task Force, Groves Conference on Marriage and the Family

Chair: Eleanor D. Macklin

Epidemiology and Public Health

Chair: Richard H. Needle

Anne H. Coulson
Jean E. Veevers
Bruce Voeller

Education and Prevention

Chair: Jeri Hepworth

G. Mary Bourne
Sandra L. Caron
Kenneth R. Davis
John L. McAdoo
Ronald M. Moglia
Nelwyn B. Moore
Timothy M. Sankary
Mary Lee Tatum
Robert H. Walsh
Anne Welbourne-Moglia

Human Services and Treatment

Chair: Kay B. Tiblier

Constance Avery-Clark
Ira J. Bates
Seldon Illick
Andrew M. Mattison
Irene T. Morin
John S. Rolland
Mary Jane Van Meter
Gillian Walker

Public Policy

Chair: Elaine A. Anderson

Diane Beeson
Theresa L. Crenshaw
Douglas A. Feldman
Mark R. Ginsberg
Carol Levine
Robert M. Rice
Virginia Sibbison
Marvin B. Sussman
Steven M. Vincent
Deborah Weinstein

Societal Implications

Chair: D. Bruce Carter

John H. Curtis
Clive M. Davis
David McWhirter
James W. Ramey
Stephanie A. Sanders
Jean R. Smith
Louise Tyrer

Anderson, Elaine A., PhD, Associate Professor, Department of Family and Community Development, University of Maryland, College Park, Maryland.

Avery-Clark, Constance, PhD, Research and Clinical Associate/Director of Continuing Education, Masters and Johnson Institute, St. Louis, Missouri.

Bates, Ira J., PhD, MPH, Director of Educational Services, National Hospice Organization, Arlington, Virginia.

Beeson, Diane, PhD, Associate Professor, Department of Sociology and Social Services, California State University, Hayward, California.

Bourne, G. Mary, ACSW, President and Director of Training, Minnesota Institute of Family Dynamics, Minneapolis, Minnesota.

Caron, Sandra L., PhD, Assistant Professor, School of Human Development, University of Maine, Orono, Maine.

Carter, D. Bruce, PhD, Associate Professor, Department of Psychology, Syracuse University, Syracuse, New York.

Coulson, Anne, Research Epidemiologist and Senior Lecturer, Division of Epidemiology, School of Public Health, University of California, Los Angeles, California.

Crenshaw, Theresa L., MD, Director, Crenshaw Clinic, San Diego, California.

Curtis, John H., PhD, Professor, Department of Sociology and Anthropology, Valdosta State College, Valdosta, Georgia.

Davis, Clive M., PhD, Associate Professor, Department of Psychology, Syracuse University, Syracuse, New York.

Davis, Kenneth R., ACSW, Lecturer, Departments of Ethnic Studies and Sociology, University of California, Hayward, California.

Feldman, Douglas A., PhD, Chair, AIDS and Anthropology Task Force, American Anthropological Association, Kew Gardens, New York.

Ginsberg, Mark R., PhD, Executive Director, American Association for Marriage and Family Therapy, Washington, D.C.

Hepworth, Jeri, PhD, Assistant Professor and Director, Behavioral Sciences, Department of Family Medicine, University of Connecticut Health Center, Hartford, Connecticut.

Illick, Selden, ACSW, Princeton Psychological Associates, Princeton, New Jersey.

Levine, Carol, Executive Director, Citizens Commission on AIDS for New York City and Northern New Jersey, New York.

Macklin, Eleanor D., PhD, Associate Professor and Director, Marriage and Family Therapy Program, Department of Child, Family and Community Studies, Syracuse University, Syracuse, New York.

Mattison, Andrew M., MSW, PhD, Assistant Clinical Professor, Department of Family and Community Medicine, School of Medicine, University of California, San Diego, California.

McAdoo, John L., PhD, Associate Professor, School of Social Work and Community Planning, University of Maryland at Baltimore, Baltimore, Maryland.

McWhirter, David, MD, Associate Clinical Professor, Department of Psychiatry, School of Medicine, University of California, San Diego, California.

Moglia, Ronald, EdD, Professor and Director, Human Sexuality Program, Department of Health Education, New York University, New York, New York.

Moore, Nelwyn B., PhD, Professor, Department of Home Economics, Southwest Texas State University, San Marcos, Texas.

Morin, Irene T., LCSW, Service Supervisor, North Baltimore Center, Baltimore, Maryland.

Needle, Richard H., PhD, Professor, Department of Family Social Science and School of Public Health, University of Minnesota, Minneapolis, Minnesota.

Ramey, James W., PhD, Former Chair, AIDS Task Force, Society for the Scientific Study of Sex, Philadelphia, Pennsylvania.

Rice, Robert M., PhD, Executive Vice President, Family Service America, Milwaukee, Wisconsin.

Rolland, John S., MD, Assistant Professor, Department of Psychiatry, School of Medicine, Yale University and Medical Director, Center for Illness in Families, New Haven, Connecticut.

Sanders, Stephanie, A., PhD, Science Assistant to the Director, Kinsey Institute for Research in Sex, Gender, and Reproduction, Indiana University, Bloomington, Indiana.

Sankary, Timothy M., MD, MPH, Director, More-Health Institute, San Francisco, California.

Sibbison, Virginia, PhD, Executive Director, Welfare Research, Inc., Albany, New York.

Smith, Jean R., MDiv, Associate Rector, Trinity Church, Princeton, New Jersey.

Sussman, Marvin B., PhD, UNIDEL Professor of Human Behavior, College of Human Resources, University of Delaware, Newark, Delaware.

Tatum, Mary Lee, MEd, Family Life/Sexuality Educator, Falls Church Public Schools, Falls Church, Virginia.

Tiblier, Kay B., PhD, Associate Clinical Professor, School of Nursing, University of California, San Francisco, California.

Tyrer, Louise, MD, Vice President for Medical Affairs, Planned Parenthood Federation of America, Inc., New York, New York.

Van Meter, Mary Jane S., PhD, Associate Professor, Department of Sociology, Wayne State University, Detroit, Michigan.

Veevers, Jean E., PhD, Professor, Department of Sociology, University of Victoria, British Columbia, Canada.

Vincent, Steven M., PhD, Psychology and Outpatient Counseling Center, St. Cloud Hospital, St. Cloud, Minnesota.

Voeller, Bruce, PhD, President, Mariposa Foundation, Topanza, California.

Walker, Gillian, ACSW, Co-Director, AIDS Project, Ackerman Institute for Family Therapy, New York, New York.

Walsh, Robert H., PhD, Professor and Chairperson, Department of Sociology, Illinois State University, Normal, Illinois.

Weinstein, Deborah, MSW, Former Executive Director, Society for the Scientific Study of Sex, Philadelphia, Pennsylvania.

Welbourne-Moglia, Ann, PhD, Former Executive Director, Sex Information and Education Council of the United States; consultant and psychologist in private practice, New York, New York.

National Coalition on AIDS and Families: Goal Statement and General Principles

GOAL STATEMENT

The National Coalition on AIDS and Families is a working association of organizations and professionals concerned with the impact of the AIDS epidemic on families. Recognizing both the strengths and needs of families, and acknowledging the diverse forms which families may assume, it advocates for families by (a) educating organizations, human service and family professionals, and the public; (b) influencing public policy; (c) serving as an information resource; (d) stimulating research; and (e) providing a forum for professional networking.

GENERAL PRINCIPLES

- AIDS affects families and not just the individual who contracts the disease.
- The family plays a key role in education, prevention, and attitude change regarding AIDS.
- The family must be seen as the unit of care in the treatment of AIDS. Families need to be educated regarding this role and be provided the support required in order to be effective.
- The impact on the family continues beyond the illness and death of the infected member.
- Special attention must be given to the needs of low-income families and minority families because these families, with multiple burdens, suffer severely from the AIDS epidemic.
- The impact of the AIDS epidemic on families, and the reaction of families, will vary with ethnicity, religion, race, and social class.
- Efforts must be made to reduce the stigma, discrimination, and isolation of families with an HIV-infected member.

269

- Preventative and educational efforts must be rational, pragmatic, and supportive of healthy sexuality.
- Decisions regarding the psychosocial aspects of prevention and treatment must be based on solid theory and research.
- Social policy regarding AIDS must recognize and respond to the strengths and needs of families.

Co-Chairs:

Sandra Caron, Eleanor Macklin, and John Rolland.

Steering Committee:

Elaine Anderson, Diane Beeson, Mary Bourne, Bruce Carter, Jeri Hepworth, Edward Kain, Richard Needle, Lori Rogovin, John Rolland, Michael Shernoff, Kay Tiblier, and Gillian Walker.

Address:

c/o Marriage and Family Therapy Program
College for Human Development
Syracuse University
Syracuse, NY 13244-1250
(315) 443-3023

Index

Abortion, 217
Abstinence, sexual, 49-50
Ackerman Institute for Family Therapy,
    AIDS Project, 67,83,127,262
Acquired immune deficiency syndrome.
    See AIDS
Acquired immune deficiency
    syndrome-related conditions *See*
    ARC
Adolescents
    with AIDS, 28,219
    AIDS education programs for, 57,169
    AIDS epidemiology among, 28-29
    drug use, 28
    safer sex practices, 74
    sex education for, 44,46,70-72,168-171
    sexual abstinence, 49
    sexually activity, 49,170-171
Africa, HIV epidemiology, 5,14
AIDS (acquired immune deficiency
    syndrome)
    behavioral factors, 16,48
        risk reduction practices, 217-220,227.
        See also Safer sex
        social policy regarding, 217-218,227
    biopsychosocial stages, 105-115
        AIDS diagnosis, 110-113
        ARC diagnosis, 109-110
        bereavement/reorganization, 113-115
        seropositivity, 106-109
        "worried well", 105-106
    deaths from, 5,14,45
    definition, 14
    diagnostic criteria, 133
    drug treatment, 31-32,110-111
        azidothymidine, 32,111,150-152,164,
        202
    epidemiology. *See* Epidemiology, of
        AIDS

first reported cases, 4
health care. *See* Health care,
    AIDS-related
high-risk populations. *See also* Bisexual
    men; Homosexual(s); IV drug users
    AIDS education programs for, 44
    mandatory HIV antibody testing,
    140-141
    psychosocial needs, 95-105
incidence, 4-5,13-14,31,45
    projected, 146
    worldwide, 14,230
information sources, 31,67-68,93,
    241-264. *See also* Educational
    programs, for AIDS prevention
    for adolescents, 251
    for adult education, 251-252
    audio-video materials, 260-262
    for families and caregivers, 257-259
    historical, 242-244
    regarding hospice care, 249-251
    media-related, 43-44,247-248
    medical, 248-249
    for minorities, 70
    newsletters, 259-260
    nutritional, 249
    organizations, 262-264
    periodicals, 259-260
    political, 246-247
    resource list, 255-264
    sociological, 244-246
media coverage, 43-44,60,217
    in Great Britain, 247-248
    sensationalism in, 137-138
medical care. *See* Health care,
    AIDS-related
medical costs. *See* Health care,
    AIDS-related, costs
medical progression, 110-113

     271

2/19